COMMUNICATING CLEARLY ABOUT MEDICINES

PROCEEDINGS OF A WORKSHOP

Joe Alper, *Rapporteur*

Roundtable on Health Literacy

Board on Population Health and Public Health Practice

Health and Medicine Division

The National Academies of
SCIENCES · ENGINEERING · MEDICINE

THE NATIONAL ACADEMIES PRESS
Washington, DC
www.nap.edu

THE NATIONAL ACADEMIES PRESS 500 Fifth Street, NW Washington, DC 20001

This activity was supported by contracts between the National Academy of Sciences and AbbVie Inc.; Aetna Foundation; Agency for Healthcare Research and Quality (HHSP23337024); American Dental Association; Bristol-Myers Squibb; East Bay Community Foundation (Kaiser Permanente); Eli Lilly and Company; Health Literacy Media; Health Literacy Partners; Health Resources and Services Administration (HHSH25034011T); Humana; Institute for Healthcare Advancement; Merck Sharp & Dohme Corp.; National Institutes of Health (HHSN26300054); National Library of Medicine; Northwell Health; Office of Disease Prevention and Health Promotion (HHSP23337043); and UnitedHealth Group. Any opinions, findings, conclusions, or recommendations expressed in this publication do not necessarily reflect the views of any organization or agency that provided support for the project.

International Standard Book Number-13: 978-0-309-46185-6
International Standard Book Number-10: 0-309-46185-5
Digital Object Identifier: https://doi.org/10.17226/24814

Additional copies of this publication are available for sale from the National Academies Press, 500 Fifth Street, NW, Keck 360, Washington, DC 20001; (800) 624-6242 or (202) 334-3313; http://www.nap.edu.

Printed in the United States of America.

Suggested citation: National Academies of Sciences, Engineering, and Medicine. 2017. *Communicating clearly about medicines: Proceedings of a workshop*. Washington, DC: The National Academies Press. doi: https://doi.org/10.17226/24814.

The National Academies of

SCIENCES • ENGINEERING • MEDICINE

The **National Academy of Sciences** was established in 1863 by an Act of Congress, signed by President Lincoln, as a private, nongovernmental institution to advise the nation on issues related to science and technology. Members are elected by their peers for outstanding contributions to research. Dr. Marcia McNutt is president.

The **National Academy of Engineering** was established in 1964 under the charter of the National Academy of Sciences to bring the practices of engineering to advising the nation. Members are elected by their peers for extraordinary contributions to engineering. Dr. C. D. Mote, Jr., is president.

The **National Academy of Medicine** (formerly the Institute of Medicine) was established in 1970 under the charter of the National Academy of Sciences to advise the nation on medical and health issues. Members are elected by their peers for distinguished contributions to medicine and health. Dr. Victor J. Dzau is president.

The three Academies work together as the **National Academies of Sciences, Engineering, and Medicine** to provide independent, objective analysis and advice to the nation and conduct other activities to solve complex problems and inform public policy decisions. The National Academies also encourage education and research, recognize outstanding contributions to knowledge, and increase public understanding in matters of science, engineering, and medicine.

Learn more about the National Academies of Sciences, Engineering, and Medicine at **www.nationalacademies.org**.

The National Academies of

SCIENCES · ENGINEERING · MEDICINE

Consensus Study Reports published by the National Academies of Sciences, Engineering, and Medicine document the evidence-based consensus on the study's statement of task by an authoring committee of experts. Reports typically include findings, conclusions, and recommendations based on information gathered by the committee and the committee's deliberations. Each report has been subjected to a rigorous and independent peer-review process and it represents the position of the National Academies on the statement of task.

Proceedings published by the National Academies of Sciences, Engineering, and Medicine chronicle the presentations and discussions at a workshop, symposium, or other event convened by the National Academies. The statements and opinions contained in proceedings are those of the participants and are not endorsed by other participants, the planning committee, or the National Academies.

For information about other products and activities of the National Academies, please visit www.nationalacademies.org/about/whatwedo.

PLANNING COMMITTEE ON COMMUNICATING CLEARLY ABOUT MEDICINE[1]

IRENE Z. CHAN, Deputy Director, Division of Medication Error Prevention and Analysis, U.S. Food and Drug Administration

TERRY DAVIS, Professor of Medicine and Pediatrics, Louisiana State University Health Sciences Center

JAMES (JAY) DUHIG, Head, Risk Communication and Behavioral Systems, Office of Patient Safety, AbbVie Inc.

JOAN GUTHRIE MEDLEN, Training Development Specialist, Office of Adult Abuse Prevention and Investigations, Oregon Department of Human Services; and President, Medlen Consulting, LLC

LAURIE MYERS, Global Health Literacy Director, Merck Sharp & Dohme Corp.

H. SHONNA YIN, Assistant Professor of Pediatrics and Population Health, New York University School of Medicine and Bellevue Hospital Center

[1] The National Academies of Sciences, Engineering, and Medicine's planning committees are solely responsible for organizing the workshop, identifying topics, and choosing speakers. The responsibility for the published Proceedings of a Workshop rests with the workshop rapporteur and the institution.

ROUNDTABLE ON HEALTH LITERACY[1]

[1] The National Academies of Sciences, Engineering, and Medicine's forums and roundtables do not issue, review, or approve individual documents. The responsibility for the published Proceedings of a Workshop rests with the workshop rapporteur and the institution.

MICHAEL PAASCHE-ORLOW, Professor of Medicine, Boston University School of Medicine
TERRI ANN PARNELL, Principal and Founder, Health Literacy Partners
KIM PARSON, Strategic Consultant, Proactive Care Strategies, Humana
KAVITA PATEL, Managing Director for Clinical Transformation and Delivery, The Brookings Institution
ANDREW PLEASANT, Senior Director for Health Literacy and Research, Canyon Ranch Institute
LINDSEY A. ROBINSON, Thirteenth District Trustee, American Dental Association
STACEY ROSEN, Associate Professor of Cardiology, Hofstra Northwell Health School of Medicine and Vice President, Women's Health, The Katz Institute for Women's Health
RIMA RUDD, Senior Lecturer on Health Literacy, Education, and Policy, Harvard T.H. Chan School of Public Health
STEVEN RUSH, Director, Health Literacy Innovations, UnitedHealth Group
MICHAEL VILLAIRE, Chief Executive Officer, Institute for Healthcare Advancement
EARNESTINE WILLIS, Kellner Professor in Pediatrics, Medical College of Wisconsin
MICHAEL WOLF, Professor, Medicine and Learning Sciences, Associate Division Chief, Research Division of General Internal Medicine, Feinberg School of Medicine, Northwestern University
WINSTON WONG, Medical Director, Community Benefit, Disparities Improvement, and Quality Initiatives, Kaiser Permanente

Consultant

RUTH PARKER, Professor of Medicine, Pediatrics, and Public Health, Emory University School of Medicine

Health and Medicine Division Staff

LYLA HERNANDEZ, Senior Program Officer
MELISSA FRENCH, Program Officer
ALEXIS WOJTOWICZ, Senior Program Assistant
ROSE MARIE MARTINEZ, Senior Board Director, Board on Population Health and Public Health Practice

Reviewers

This Proceedings of a Workshop was reviewed in draft form by individuals chosen for their diverse perspectives and technical expertise. The purpose of this independent review is to provide candid and critical comments that will assist the National Academies of Sciences, Engineering, and Medicine in making each published proceedings as sound as possible and to ensure that it meets the institutional standards for quality, objectivity, evidence, and responsiveness to the charge. The review comments and draft manuscript remain confidential to protect the integrity of the process.

We thank the following individuals for their review of this proceedings:

SUZANNE BAKKEN, Columbia University
SHARON E. BARRETT, Association of Clinicians for the Underserved
CATHRYN GUNTHER, Merck Sharp & Dohme Corp.
ALICE HOROWITZ, University of Maryland School of Public Health

Although the reviewers listed above provided many constructive comments and suggestions, they were not asked to endorse the content of the proceedings nor did they see the final draft before its release. The review of this proceedings was overseen by **Hugh H. Tilson,** University of North Carolina at Chapel Hill. He was responsible for making certain that an independent examination of this proceedings was carried out in accordance with standards of the National Academies and that all review comments were carefully considered. Responsibility for the final content rests entirely with the rapporteur and the National Academies.

Acknowledgments

The sponsors of the National Academies of Sciences, Engineering, and Medicine's Roundtable on Health Literacy made it possible to plan and conduct the workshop on communicating clearly about medicines, which this Proceedings of a Workshop summarizes. Federal sponsors included the Agency for Healthcare Research and Quality, Health Resources and Services Administration, National Institutes of Health, National Library of Medicine, and Office of Disease Prevention and Health Promotion at the U.S. Department of Health and Human Services. Non-federal sponsorship was provided by AbbVie Inc.; Aetna Foundation; American Dental Association; Bristol-Myers Squibb; East Bay Community Foundation (Kaiser Permanente); Eli Lilly and Company; Health Literacy Media; Health Literacy Partners; Humana; Institute for Healthcare Advancement; Merck Sharp & Dohme Corp.; Northwell Health; and UnitedHealth Group.

The roundtable would like to thank each of the speakers, reactors, and panel moderators for their time and effort. Speakers, reactors, and moderators were, in alphabetical order, Irene Chan, Donna Horn, Ed Israelski, Brian Jack, Charles Lee, Darvece A. Monson, Dan Morrow, Laurie Myers, Terri Ann Parnell, Bobbie Reed, Heather Rennie, Bernard Rosof, Caleb Sexton, William Shrank, Steve Sparks, Elisabeth Walther, Michael Wolf, and H. Shonna Yin.

Contents

Boxes and Figures

BOXES

FIGURES

Acronyms and Abbreviations

AAMI	Association for the Advancement of Medical Instrumentation
AHRQ	Agency for Healthcare Research and Quality
ANSI	American National Standards Institute
EHR	electronic health record
FDA	U.S. Food and Drug Administration
FFS	fee-for-service
HCAHPS	Hospital Consumer Assessment of Healthcare Providers and Systems
HHS	U.S. Department of Health and Human Services
IEC	International Electrotechnical Commission
ISO	International Organization for Standardization
NVS	Newest Vital Sign
PEMAT	Patient Education Materials Assessment Tool
Project RED	Reengineered Discharge Program
QR	Quick Response

UMS	Universal Medication Schedule
UPMC	University of Pittsburgh Medical Center
USP	U.S. Pharmacopeia

1

Introduction and Workshop Overview[1]

Research conducted over the past two decades has shown that poor patient understanding of medication instructions is an important contributor to the more than 1 million medication errors and adverse drug events that lead to office and emergency room visits, hospitalizations, and even death (Bates et al., 1995; Budnitz and Layde, 2007; IOM, 2007; Sarkar et al., 2011; Vrijens et al., 2012). Patients who have limited literacy skills, who have multiple comorbidities, and who are elderly face the greatest risk, and limited literacy skills are significantly associated with inadequate understanding and use of prescription instructions and precautions (Davis et al., 2006a,b; Persell et al., 2007; Wolf et al., 2006). The Agency for Healthcare Research and Quality notes that only 12 percent of U.S. adults have proficient health literacy that allows them to interpret a prescription label correctly (AHRQ, 2014).

One cause for patient misunderstanding is that physicians often fail to communicate important elements of medication use when prescribing a new medication (Tarn et al., 2006, 2013). Confusing medication labels, a topic the Roundtable on Health Literacy has tackled previously (IOM, 2008; Wolf et al., 2006), and polypharmacy associated with patients having complex disorders or multiple chronic illnesses (Fialová and Onder, 2009;

[1] The planning committee's role was limited to planning the workshop, and the Proceedings of a Workshop was prepared by the workshop rapporteur as a factual summary of what occurred at the workshop. Statements, recommendations, and opinions expressed are those of individual presenters and participants, and are not endorsed or verified by the National Academies of Sciences, Engineering, and Medicine, as they should not be construed as reflecting any group consensus.

BOX 1-1
Statement of Task

An ad hoc committee will plan and conduct a 1-day public workshop that will feature invited presentations and discussion of the role and challenges regarding clarity of communication on medication. Potential areas of focus include use of health literacy principles to address clarity of materials, decision aids, and other supportive tools and technologies regarding risks, benefits, alternatives, and health plan coverage. The committee will define the specific topics to be addressed, develop the agenda, select and invite speakers and other participants, and moderate the discussions. A summary of the presentations and discussion at the workshop will be prepared by a designated rapporteur in accordance with institutional guidelines.

Koper et al., 2013) also contribute to poor patient understanding of how to take medications properly.

Given the importance of health literacy to the proper use of medications, and the apparent lack of progress in improving medication adherence (NCPIE, 2013), the Roundtable on Health Literacy formed an ad hoc committee to plan and conduct a 1-day public workshop that featured invited presentations and discussion of the role and challenges regarding clarity of communication on medication. The Statement of Task for the committee (see Box 1-1) cited potential areas of focus to include using health literacy principles to address clarity of materials, decision aids, and other supportive tools and technologies regarding risks, benefits, alternatives, and health plan coverage. The goal of the workshop, said Bernard Rosof, chief executive officer of the Quality in Healthcare Advisory Group and roundtable chair, was to "contribute to efforts to communicate clearly by exploring the research that is currently ongoing and highlighting efforts to promote better communication." In his introduction to the workshop, Rosof said there is a good reason for the roundtable to revisit the topic of health literacy as it pertains to the proper use of medication. "Medications, of course, are a vital component of health care and health care delivery, but when they are used incorrectly they can result in poor outcomes, injury, and often, death," said Rosof. "Research has shown that almost half of all patients misunderstand one or more of their dosage instructions and slightly more than half misunderstand one or more warnings related to their medication. This misunderstanding does not necessarily reflect a failure on the part of patients or patients' families or caregivers, but rather on the rest of us in the health care system, who fail to provide information clearly and simply and take the time." He added that communicating about medications with regard to risks, benefits, and adherence has the potential to greatly improve patient understanding, encouragement, and outcomes.

Rosof explained that the workshop included only one presentation on populations with limited English proficiency not because the roundtable or workshop planning committee failed to recognize the needs of these populations. Rather, this workshop focused primarily on materials in English because the U.S. Food and Drug Administration's regulations governing drug-related materials focus on English-language speakers and because most of the research in this area has been centered on English speakers.

ORGANIZATION OF THE PROCEEDINGS

The workshop (see Appendix A for the agenda) was organized by an independent planning committee in accordance with the procedures of the National Academies of Sciences, Engineering, and Medicine. The planning committee's members were Irene Chan, Terry Davis, James Duhig, Joan Guthrie Medlen, Laurie Myers, and H. Shonna Yin. This publication summarizes the workshop's presentations and discussions, and it highlights some lessons, practical strategies, and needs and opportunities discussed by individual workshop participants for applying the principles of health literacy to the task of helping individuals understand how to use the medications they take. Chapter 2 provides the patient perspective on the challenge of understanding and following medication instructions. Chapter 3 describes the current landscape of research on written communications and various approaches to designing medication-related materials at a level appropriate for patients and caregivers. Chapter 4 presents several case studies illustrating how research findings are translated into practice. Chapter 5 discusses the future of health-literate design with regard to medication materials, and Chapter 6 recounts the roundtable members' reflections on the day.

In accordance with the policies of the National Academies, the workshop did not attempt to establish any conclusions or recommendations about needs and future directions, focusing instead on issues identified by individual speakers and workshop participants. The proceedings should not be construed as reflecting any group consensus. In addition, the organizing committee's role was limited to planning the workshop. The workshop proceedings was prepared by workshop rapporteur Joe Alper as a factual account of what occurred at the workshop.

2

Patient and Caregiver Perspectives[1]

The workshop's first panel session aimed to provide some understanding of how patients and caregivers struggle with understanding medication instructions, particularly when patients require multiple drugs to treat their conditions. The three members of the panel were Bobbie Reed, the mother and caregiver of a kidney transplant recipient who also serves as the Pennsylvania Kidney Advocacy Committee Liaison for the National Kidney Foundation;[2] Caleb Sexton, a patient with psoriatic disease who is also an advocate with the National Psoriasis Foundation[3] and a designer who focuses on health literacy technology research and human-centered design; and Darvece Monson, a nurse, patient with chronic kidney disease waiting for a kidney transplant, and founder of the advocacy organization More Than Your Kidneys.[4] Terri Ann Parnell, principal partner and founder of Health Literacy Partners, moderated the panel session and the open discussion that followed the panelists' remarks.

[1] This section is based on the presentations by Bobbie Reed, the mother and caregiver of a kidney transplant recipient and the Pennsylvania Kidney Advocacy Committee Liaison for the National Kidney Foundation; Caleb Sexton, a patient with psoriatic arthritis, an advocate with the National Psoriasis Foundation, and a designer who focuses on health literacy technology research and human-centered design; and Darvece Monson, a nurse, patient with chronic kidney disease waiting for a kidney transplant, and founder of the advocacy organization More Than Your Kidneys. The statements are not endorsed or verified by the National Academies of Sciences, Engineering, and Medicine.

[2] See https://www.kidney.org (accessed July 25, 2017).

[3] See https://www.psoriasis.org (accessed July 25, 2017).

[4] See http://www.morethanyourkidneys.org (accessed July 25, 2017).

To start the conversation, Parnell asked the panelists to share one or two lessons learned from their overall experiences with medication communication. Reed, whose son received a kidney transplant, said the biggest difficulty for her with regard to managing her son's medications was how suddenly she had to take charge. When she and her son were in training for home hemodialysis, she was linked to a pharmacy whose specialty was dialysis patients and which managed all of her son's medication. That pharmacy, she said, provided a schedule of when her son was to take the various medications he was prescribed and delivered those medications to their house automatically. However, access to that specialty pharmacy ended once her son received his new kidney and suddenly, she said, it seemed that she was at her neighborhood pharmacy every day, picking up one medication after another. Soon, though, she discovered that her pharmacy also offered a specialty service that provided a nurse case manager and around-the-clock access to a customer service representative for no charge. This specialty service coordinated all of her son's medication so that she only had to make one or two trips per month to the pharmacy to pick up his prescriptions.

To help make her job easier still, Reed developed a spreadsheet that denoted which medications her son needed to take at what times and to keep track of the number of pills on hand. This spreadsheet, which she faxes to the nurse case manager, serves two purposes, she explained. First, it lets the pharmacy and her son's doctors know that he is adhering to his medication plan, and second, it alerts the pharmacy as to when refills are needed, which enables the pharmacy to contact her son's care team and the transplant center clinic to arrange for those refills, taking the burden for doing so off her. "That was very crucial and has helped me tremendously," said Reed, who suggested that this type of mechanism should be adopted for all patients requiring multiple medications. "When I took [the spreadsheet] to the specialty pharmacy, they said they did not have anything like it and that it was an ingenious idea." In fact, the pharmacy has now adopted it as a standard part of its protocol. She noted that the responsibility for adhering to a medication plan still rests with the patient and caregivers, but it does make managing the process easier. She also remarked that the specialty pharmacy idea is a great one that needs to better promoted. "I just happened to fall upon it one day when I was at the grocery store and saw a sign that read, 'Did you know about our specialty pharmacy services?'"

Sexton, who has been dealing with the life-changing experience of having psoriatic disease for the past 10 years, agreed with Reed that services such as specialty pharmacies can play an important role in providing patients with a better foundation for understanding their medications. Such services can help patients learn how to communicate the issues that can arise when someone takes multiple medications and has to deal with multiple comorbidities associated with their medical issues. He called for the medical system to provide patients with information about the ecosystems that exist to provide long-term support outside of the medical office. Wishing that he had received that kind of information 10 years ago, he noted the existence today of organizations such as the National Psoriasis Foundation and social media networks that are available to help patients better understand their conditions and better communicate with their health care providers. In his case, being put on systemic chemotherapy drugs and biologics and having creams to put on was terrifying at first. Nobody told him what these various medications did and how they might interact to produce side effects, and nobody told him that the effects of these medications were something he would have to endure to get better.

Speaking from her perspective as both a nurse and a hemodialysis patient, Monson said a greater emphasis is needed on communicating with patients about toxicity, side effects, and adverse reactions. "The patient population generally does not understand the difference," said Monson. Thanks to her nursing experience, she said, she has been able to reduce significantly the opportunity for medication error to occur, but she doubted that she would have been so successful without that experience. She also noted that while she is young, mobile, and active, the majority of renal patients are elderly and immobile, and many are not cognitively aware or able to communicate effectively.

When she was first diagnosed with kidney failure, she was put on 14 medications, and perhaps not surprisingly, she experienced complications resulting from taking multiple medications. One night, about 6 weeks into her new life as a renal failure patient, she awoke coughing and could not stop. At first, she could not figure out why, but then her "nurse light clicked" and she realized that her coughing was a side effect of taking four different antihypertensive agents. "That is going to happen, but someone else in my situation does not know that. It was not printed on the medication to look for this side effect," said Monson. She polled her fellow patients at her local dialysis center and found out that 87 percent of them did not know about this type of medication complication. She also noted that most of her fellow dialysis patients were coming from nursing homes and acute care centers and were drained by the experience of traveling to the center and undergoing dialysis. Showing someone in that condition a video explaining their medications and expecting them to develop a better understanding is unrealistic, she said. "We have to consider that and come up with better ways to communicate effectively the detriments," said Monson.

Before asking the panelists to answer another question, Parnell recounted some of the words the panelists used in a phone call prior to the workshop to describe their experiences communicating with care team members about medications: intimidated, barriers, overwhelmed, terrifying, confusions, side effects, statistical information to help with risk and benefit, challenging, hard, discouraging, put off, and taken aback. "I found it overwhelming to hear all of those terms used to describe communicating about medications," said Parnell. She then asked the panelists to state the one question they wish their prescribing clinicians would ask them when prescribing medications or changing a medication regimen. Sexton said he wanted to be asked what his biggest fear was, for in his mind this would have conveyed empathy regarding the challenges he would face and a willingness to help him, both then and in the future, deal with the unknowns regarding the many medications he would be taking for the rest of his life.

Parnell commented at that point that the idea of asking a patient about their fears was a revelation to her. "I thought I did a pretty good job over the years, always open to learning," she said. "I would ask, 'What is your typical day like, do you think you will be able to do this, who fills your medications, are you able to get them?' I would ask many questions, but never did I ask, 'What is your biggest fear or what is your biggest concern?'"

Reed then recounted an experience she had at a pretransplant surgery visit with her son's surgeon. The surgeon reviewed the medications her son would be taking after receiving his transplant, and when she asked the surgeon about a substitute for one of the immunosuppressants in this regimen—she had already gone to the literature to familiarize herself with the drugs used to treat her son's condition—he completely shut her down. The protocol was set, he told her, and he did not want to consider any modifications. That response, she said, was discouraging because it dismissed all of the research she had done proactively and discounted the initiative she had shown to learn more about the drugs her son would be taking. A better response, said Reed, would have been to say that her suggestion was interesting and that he would check it out.

Monson replied that she would like to be asked what she, as an individual, is experiencing that seems out of place, but that may or may not indicate something is wrong. For example, she said, she is very strict about her fluids compliance and is doing well with regard to the symptoms she would show if her disease was progressing. The result, she said, is that her clinician cuts her visits short without asking if something new is going on in her life. She noted that while her nursing background helps her notice symptoms not associated with her kidney disease that are likely related to the drugs she is taking, that is not true for most people. She suggested that people keep a diary to track how they feel throughout the day and of any unusual feelings or symptoms they are experiencing. They can then use that diary as a way of advocating for themselves with their physicians.

Sexton agreed that physicians should encourage their patients with chronic conditions to keep a journal, whether on paper or using an enabling technology, as a means of creating a two-way flow of information that would ultimately help the physician respond to the specific needs of individual patients. He noted that when patients with life-altering chronic illnesses visit their physicians every few months, they are asked generic questions such as "What happened in the past 3 months?" Without some type of journal, few patients would be able to answer that question in any meaningful way. "It is critical that we have a better understanding of the context and lived experiences of our patients by being able to enable that kind of data capture and make it meaningful so that both the care provider and patient can better manage their care more effectively and more efficiently in ways that really look at what is going on in their life," said Sexton. "Are they having dietary issues? Are they having more stress? What is going on outside of being in this room? What is outside of the medical record that we can pull up on our electronic health record (EHR) systems?" Sexton added that this type of patient-recorded information could help physicians identify side effect issues or life events that make compliance difficult.

Next, Parnell asked the panelists for their ideas on what clinicians can do to enhance communication, whether written or oral. One suggestion Reed had specific for kidney dialysis patients, which she heard from her son's posttransplant coordinator, is for there to be multiple education sessions for patients during which they would gradually learn about their medications. Her son's transplant coordinator told her that too many patients come to her unprepared to manage the multiple drugs they require after a transplant because the dialysis centers have previously taken care of everything and the patients never learn to take charge of their medications on their own. "By the time they get to [the coordinator], having got a kidney transplant, she finds that those patients are losing their organs or they are going into rejection simply because they are telling her that they cannot manage their medications. They do not know how to take them or when they should take them." Parnell remarked that health literacy experts talk about conveying information in chunks, of giving them two or three key points and then building on those points. Reed agreed that type of approach would help patients take ownership of their particular situation and empower them to do even more down the road.

Monson suggested that everyone on the health care team needs to be proactive about being partners with their patients and encouraging them to ask questions and talk about what they are experiencing on a day-to-day basis. For example, as a 34-year-old when she was first diagnosed, she was still ovulating and the many medications she was taking were interfering with her menstrual cycle. She knew something was wrong, but because the majority of patients on dialysis are elderly, nobody at the dialysis center even thought to consider how the 14 drugs she was taking would affect her menstrual cycle. It was only through a close relationship she developed with the pharmacist on her care team that the two of them were able to figure out what was happening and change how she was being treated. Now, she said, she is participating in four research studies aimed at understanding more about how the typical drug regimen for kidney dialysis patients interacts in a younger woman. What worries Monson is that not everyone can communicate as well as she can or has the background that she does to know to pay attention to things that seem out of the ordinary and report them to their care team members.

Reed noted a book, *The Patient Will See You Now*, that helped her communicate effectively with her son's physicians. This book talks about how to set expectations and what to expect from care team members. "It was well worth reading in terms of communicating, trying to get your point across, and getting people to do what you want them to do," said Reed.

For her final question to the panelists, Parnell asked them for one innovative solution to enhance medication communication. Both Reed and Monson nominated the need for funding to assist with medication and better information about different funding mechanisms. Reed, for example, worries that her 26-year-old son will lose Medicare coverage for his medications, which he needs to take for the rest of his life, after 36 months. Monson noted that every pharmaceutical company has options to help people with medication costs, but many people are not aware of those programs, and if they do know of them are intimidated to apply for assistance. She said that care team members need to do more to raise awareness of those assistance programs, other safety net programs, and even clinical trials that can help patients deal with the cost of their medications.

Sexton said one of the most fundamental and simple innovations would be to reframe the perspective of care providers when thinking about these long-term chronic conditions. Such a diagnosis means that patients will experience drastic changes in their lives. "It is a constant experience that has to be navigated," said Sexton, and physicians need to think about the impact of that diagnosis as more than just something that triggers office visits, but rather as a journey. He believes that thinking of these conditions in that way will change the mindset of physicians and how they think about providing care for their patients.

Sexton also noted that he has been working on technology solutions that can enable better avenues of communication between patients and clinicians and increase providers' understanding of what their patients' lives are like and the experiences that have been associated with their medical conditions. The goal of such technology solutions, he said, should be to empower patients to do something meaningful in their lives and not feel that they are stuck in a terrifying situation through which they have to suffer alone. "Even if it is as simple as designing applications that allow you to just track your metabolism or your food diary, your sleep, or your stress levels and be able to connect that back to your doctor's EHR so that whenever you come back, it is no longer those 10 generic question or those 10 generic responses. It is very specific answers and very specific questions about instances and situations in your patient's life, so you can better say, 'Maybe we need to make a pivot. Maybe this medication is not working. Maybe we should try something new.'" Such applications, said Sexton, could help create a relationship and establish two-way communication so that treating chronic conditions becomes a partnership rather than a doctor-driven dictatorship.

Reed added that it is vitally important for EHR systems to be able to communicate with one another, particularly with regard to medications. Her son, for example, cannot list all of his medications on a medical alert identification bracelet. In Pittsburgh, where her son lives, there are two major medical systems that do not share medical records. "There has to be some sort of centralized network going forward so that no matter where you are, the information is accessible," said Reed.

DISCUSSION

Terry Davis from the Louisiana State University Health Sciences Center began the discussion by recounting a story told by her research assistant, who said she was tired of the health care system thinking of her solely as a patient with type 1 diabetes who should be treated with the standard evidence-based treatment protocol and not as a 28-year-old who runs marathons, goes camping, and drinks beer with her friends. She then asked the panelists if they had any idea how to get clinicians to think beyond the standard treatment protocols and consider how individuals lead their lives. Monson replied that the only way she knows to accomplish this is for patients to take responsibility for letting their clinicians know they need to consider the human factor when developing treatment plans. "The human factor has to be the individualistic source of wellness," said Monson, who considers herself a 36-year-old marathoner, triathlete, and personal trainer, not a kidney failure patient. "Everybody focuses on my failure, but what about the other elements of my life?" she said. At one point, she recalled, she had a catheter in her heart for 7 months and was immunocompromised. "I still had to take care of my family, be a nurse, raise a child, and be a woman. How can I do that? No one ever asked me about that."

Sexton agreed with Monson and argued that while physicians have to be objective, they also need to be empathetic and aim to understand the individual, not just the patient. The best physicians consider their patients' goals and aspirations and work with their patients to create care plans to get them where they want to be. Davis added that one thing physicians can do to change their perspectives from patient to person is to ask a patient about their greatest fears, their issues, and their goals.

Jennifer Dillaha from the Arkansas Department of Health noted that many of the comments so far reflected something she observed in the early trials of drugs for HIV, which is that the factor that seemed to make the biggest different in terms of medication adherence was whether or not the patient perceived that people in the clinic cared about them. Given that, she asked the panelists if there were things they wished the people they interact with could do differently to better communicate empathy in a way that would influence how well they could adhere to their medication regimen. Reed said when she and her son went for their initial transplant evaluation, they endured an unbelievably long day in which they were overwhelmed with information. When she suggested afterward that it might be better if the transplant center could hold a series of mini-workshops at which potential patients and their caregivers could be given the same amount of information at a more reasonable pace and in a more interactive learning environment, she was shot down. Reed also noted that while her son's experience at the dialysis center was largely positive, the experience of being on the transplant waiting list was "a horrendous experience" that involved interacting with five different transplant coordinators. "I think there has to be continuity and there has to be ongoing education as opposed to a one and done deal," said Reed.

Ruth Parker from the Emory University School of Medicine asked the panelists for their thoughts on how digital technologies could be leveraged to get patients and their caregivers good, clear, actionable, health-literate information about medication. Reed has found social media, particularly Facebook, to be a starting point, although she has been unable to find any groups relating to her son's illness and the medications he has to take. She commented that people on dialysis sit in a chair multiple times per week for hours at a time, usually watching television or surfing the Internet. "That would be a perfect opportunity or an access point for you to get the information out there and ask them questions," said Reed. She also noted that some dialysis centers use a device that transmits data from a home dialysis unit to the center. Her son did not have access to that device, but it would have made her job and the clinic nurse manager's job easier.

Sexton added that social networks are crucial sources of information. These networks can be in the form of forums run by national foundations or patient support groups on Facebook or Twitter, for example. "Those kinds of forums and those support groups are so mission critical because they give you a voice and an understanding that there are other people out there like you," said Sexton. He commented that there are many digital tools and mobile phone apps available, but most are unable to integrate with an EHR system and thus cannot feed potentially useful information to providers. This is doable, however, and he noted that all of the major EHR vendors are working to develop applications that will enable their systems to access third-party datasets. As an example, he said that Humana has developed smart scales that integrate with its EHR system so that clinicians can better manage and track weight loss, which has improved outcomes. The challenge going forward, said Sexton, is to create streamlined digital ecosystems in which different components of an EHR system can exchange data among themselves and with patient-generated data as a means of increasing access to information by both the patient and the patient's care providers. Parker asked Sexton for his opinion on the use of interactive payment systems as a means of communicating about medications. Sexton said such systems are necessary and could be used to push reminders to patients and then feedback adherence data to the patient's care providers. He noted that he uses a whiteboard on which he lists when he needs to take which medication as well as setting multiple reminders on his smartphone.

Jane Grover from the American Dental Association asked the panelists if their oral health providers were informed about their medical conditions and if their medical providers asked about their oral health status. Monson said the first symptoms of her kidneys failing—the result, she believes, of the 38 pills per day she had been taking 1.5 years prior to that to treat pregnancy-induced hypertension—was a bad taste in her mouth, which affected her desire to eat. While she neglected to mention this to her physician, she did tell her dentist, who could find nothing wrong with her. She learned some 3 months later, when diagnosed with kidney failure, that the bad taste in her mouth is one of the symptoms of kidney failure. She also noted how important oral health is for a person on dialysis given how critical diet is when undergoing dialysis.

As an aside, Monson commented that dialysis centers do not allow patients to post pictures on social media, but she thinks this is a bad policy because it perpetuates the dismal image of dialysis. "We are not encouraging the idea that you can be on dialysis and have a healthy attitude."

Reed remarked that dental care was stressed throughout her son's dialysis and transplant journey, and after her son received his transplant he was informed that he would have to take antibiotics prior to any dental procedure going forward. She noted that she and her husband are proactive parents who make sure that their son has regular dental appointments as well as an annual dermatology exam because of his elevated risk of developing skin cancers as a result of the medications he takes.

Laurie Francis from the Oregon Primary Care Association commented that the remarks so far point to the convergence of patient care, human-centered design, and health literacy, and their impact on medication compliance. She then asked how to incorporate patients' lives, needs, strengths, resilience, and fears in the way the health care system approaches patients at the time of first contact. "How would it look if we met you where you are with what you are wondering about and built your care with you around your goals instead of us constantly trying to tell you how we would like you to meet our goals?" she asked the panelists. Monson agreed that meeting her where she was—a mother of a 6-year-old and an unemployed nurse who could no longer afford her medications—instead of focusing on where the medical system needed her to be would have alleviated some of the enormous pressure she was under in the months after her diagnosis. In her case, her fiancé kept her going, prodding her to go to her appointments and keep a positive attitude. She now believes she needs to be the poster child for renal disease every day. Sexton added how important it is to get the message that life goes on during difficult times. He related how much he appreciated hearing from his dermatologist that there will be hard times coming because of the multiple medications he would be taking, but that if he took care of himself life would be meaningful and not all about his illness. "The psychological effects, the social effects are so critical," said Sexton. "We miss the boat on that quite frequently." Monson agreed, which is why she named her organization More Than Your Kidneys to reflect the fact that patients need to figure out what type of life they are going to live beyond their diagnosis and that they are likely to need help from outside of the medical system to do so because most physicians are not equipped to provide that kind of advice.

Reed said she would have liked to have had a roadmap to give her of what may happen on the journey ahead. Instead, she had to continually ask questions and set her own plan into action based on what might or might not happen. Two important steps, she said, are to explain to patients what can happen if they do not adhere to their medication regimen and how they will benefit when they stay on their plan.

Wilma Alvarado-Little from Alvarado-Little Consulting said what resonated with her from the panelists' remarks was the issue of empowerment and advocating for oneself. She then asked the panelists if they had any advice for parents who have to advocate for their children. Reed replied that having a good support network is important when you have a child with a terrible disease and that there are support groups available that are geared specifically toward the parents of pediatric patients.

Robert Logan from the National Library of Medicine noted that there are medical centers in the United States that specialize in listening to a patient's life and journey stories and embrace diverse comments as a foundation of patient-centered clinical care. Logan cited the Nuka System of Care model practiced by the Southcentral Foundation in Anchorage, Alaska,[5] as an example of how innovative approaches to listening to patients also are

[5] See https://www.southcentralfoundation.com (accessed on March 31, 2017).

linked to clinical quality improvements. "Many of the things you discussed are definitely in place and are making significant clinical differences," said Logan. "I wish those places (medical centers) were the model that was used throughout the United States and in other countries around the world." Bernard Rosof concluded the discussion by recounting a comment that Donald Berwick, former administrator of the Centers for Medicare & Medicaid Services, made in a commencement address. Speaking to new graduates of Yale Medical School, Berwick told the graduates to take off their white coats and sit among their patients to get insights into what they really need to know. "That is what I think I heard today from the panel," said Rosof. He added that while technology, data, and social media are important elements to caring for patients with complex illnesses, personal involvement, concern, and communication remain key elements.

3

Approaches to Health-Literate Medication Instructions

The workshop's second panel featured three presentations on the current landscape of research on written communication and human-centered design. William Shrank, chief medical officer of the University of Pittsburgh Medical Center (UPMC) Health Plan, discussed research on written communications. Irene Chan, deputy director in the Division of Medication Error Prevention and Analysis at the U.S. Food and Drug Administration (FDA), then spoke about designing labels and labeling for patients, and Edmond Israelski, technical advisor on human factors and retired director of human factors at AbbVie Inc., addressed the use of best practice human-centered design methods in the design of medication materials. An open discussion moderated by Bernard Rosof followed the three presentations.

AN OVERVIEW OF RESEARCH ON WRITTEN COMMUNICATIONS[1]

Fifteen years ago, when William Shrank was starting a fellowship, health literacy was just becoming a topic of interest, thanks to the pioneering work of Terry Davis and Ruth Parker. "When you think about where the discussion was then and where the discussion is today, it is pretty extraordinary the amount of progress and change and to some extent, a

[1] This section is based on the presentation by William Shrank, chief medical officer of the UPMC Health Plan, and the statements are not endorsed or verified by the National Academies of Sciences, Engineering, and Medicine.

lack of coordination, but also an extraordinary amount of innovation," said Shrank. He then noted how important it is today to look at the issue of health literacy and communication about medications in the context of the rapidly changing health care landscape. In this new era of paying for quality instead of for volume, providers are taking on more financial risk, which is leading them to become more concerned than ever about what happens to patients once they leave the doctor's office. As a result, providers need to better communicate and engage with their patients. "It means that these measures that some of us have been doing research on for a long time are suddenly front and center in every primary care doctor's office with regard to how their patients are taking their medications," said Shrank.

This fundamental change, he said, creates a unique business context for a host of players in the industry to participate in efforts to improve communication with patients. Pharmacies, for example, are now partnering with health systems to support patients between visits to their doctors, and pharmacy benefits managers are creating a better infrastructure and collecting data for tracking whether patients are adhering to medication plans. Countless start-up companies are trying to find a niche in which they can support providers. The result, said Shrank, is that there is an enormous amount of attention, growth, and interest in understanding how to better communicate and support patients regarding their medication use.

Another fundamental change in health care that is germane to health literacy and medication adherence is the shift in cost sharing from employers to their employees. As a result, Shrank explained, patients are now educating themselves about price and quality like never before and are making provider choices based at least in part on such information. Patients today, he said, are looking for practices that explain more, that make their patients feel cared for, and where they believe there is some mechanism in place to help them manage their complex lives and medication regimens. "That means that anyone who cares about whether that consumer gets their care at their site or through their service sure better figure out how to communicate with that consumer," said Shrank.

Shrank then claimed there is more investment in this area today than he could have ever imagined. As an example, he explained how CVS Health, a large retail pharmacy chain with a reputation for working with and focusing on consumers, allocates substantial resources to understand what words work in terms of patient communications, what messages work, what vehicles work, and how messages should be delivered. CVS Health also works with a remarkably deep set of analytics and predictive modeling, he added, to rapidly assess what is working or not working, and continually strive to understand how to get the right intervention to the right person. "These investments are driving the way CVS communicates with patients, the words they choose, the channels that they leverage, and the way in which they are continually trying to improve," said Shrank, who formerly worked for CVS.

Health systems, including the UPMC health plan where he currently works, are also investing a significant amount of energy in figuring out how to communicate better with its providers' patients. "We have a rich, robust consumer innovation arm and have acquired probably a dozen companies specifically to help us use different kinds of technology and different kinds of data to better target and deliver the right intervention to the right patient regarding their medications or their chronic disease management," explained Shrank. The focus of this work, which now involves more than 100 employees at the UPMC health plan, is on learning internally, improving continually, and running the business as well as possible, but with a "deep and profound commitment to understanding how we communicate with our patients best to deliver the very best care we can."

One result from all of these efforts, said Shrank, is that patients may actually become overwhelmed with information. "A patient with diabetes and heart failure might be getting calls from many different sources," he said. Another issue is that while the field is investing enormous resources in this type of research, there is no collaboration among organizations. "Ultimately, there is a great deal of inefficiency here," said Shrank. "We are all studying many of these same questions, approaching them in many of the same ways, and leveraging many of the same analytics. A rising tide would lift all ships here if we were able to bring together all of these efforts, all of these resources, all of this speed, and all of this business urgency to create learning from which we all could benefit." He has argued there is a business case for sharing what we have learned and publishing results. "It does allow you to differentiate yourself from your competitors and make a clear value-driven, mission-driven argument around what you are trying to do to help support your members or your patients or your customers," said Shrank.

One important new factor is the explosion of tools to promote wellness and chronic disease. Fifteen years ago, medication labels were the only way to talk to patients about their medications. Today, a variety of tools, including online resources, mobile device apps, texting, and telephone approaches, exist for patients to learn about their medications. "This speaks to the fact that the kinds of questions we are asking and the kinds of interventions we can apply are expanding rapidly," said Shrank. He noted it would be shortsighted to focus research on any one of these approaches at the expense of the others.

In addition, he said that not only are there many tools and vehicles for sharing information, but the messages themselves can vary. Messages can focus on education or risk, and can use techniques such as behavioral economics to encourage and motivate patients. Social networks are an increasing source of information transfer and encouragement. "When you start layering all of these tools with all of these tactics, the number of permutations is quite enormous," said Shrank. As a result, researchers need to be thoughtful about not just saying one works and one does not, but instead stating which intervention is right for which specific type of patient and saying how one approach compares to the other sets of innovations. The goal, he said, is to determine how to create a cohesive, coordinated approach to bring the right intervention to the right person without being wasteful or sending too many interventions to any given person. "How do you build the right system, a comprehensive, thoughtful system that can really help patients better take their meds?" asked Shrank.

Going forward, said Shrank, the health care environment is changing faster than anyone could have imagined even a few years ago and the movement to value will continue regardless of the change in administrations. "It is now hard-wired into how government pays for care and how commercial payers are paying for care, and increasingly it is being adopted by providers as their mission to deliver better care at lower cost," he said. He predicted the result will be that the level of investment in this area will only increase, as will the need for those researchers attending this workshop to play a substantial role in refining, reforming, and encouraging the research community to play a different role in the marketplace. Researchers, he said, need to "embed themselves in a company or to partner deeply with a company that has scale, that has the ability to test and expand, that has the resources that can do things quickly. That kind of embedded approach would allow us to take into account all of the nuances, all of the different levers, all of the different approaches."

As an example of this approach, Shrank cited the work Michael Wolf did on the Universal Medical Schedule, a methodology that simplifies medication instructions for patients and their caregivers. Wolf did some foundational work with Ruth Parker, Terry Davis, and to a lesser extent himself (Shrank et al., 2010), and then worked closely with companies in the marketplace to test this approach and then scale it (Wolf et al., 2016). In closing, Shrank added that embedding this type of work in health care and commercial organizations could provide a way of funding health literacy research.

THE ROLE OF HUMAN FACTORS ENGINEERING[2]

When it comes to designing labels and labeling information,[3] what FDA hopes for is a design that translates into safe and effective use of the medications on the market by end users, including patients, caregivers, and health care providers, Chan explained. One goal of designing labels and labeling is to avoid medication error, which she defined as any preventable event that may cause or lead to inappropriate medication use or patient harm while the medication is in the control of the health care professional, patient, or provider. The key term here is prevention, she said, adding, "We are trying to prevent an event that could lead to inappropriate medication use or patient harm."

A 2007 report from the Institute of Medicine (IOM, 2007) noted that labeling and packaging issues cause 33 percent of all medication errors. This report urged FDA to use human factors analysis to improve labeling information and nomenclature. Human factors analysis, she explained, is about understanding the interactions among humans and elements of a system with the goal of optimizing human well-being and overall system performance. "Putting those concepts together—medication error prevention and human factors—we see they are interconnected," said Chan. "If we want to prevent medication errors, we have to be looking critically at human factors with the combined goal of ensuring that there is appropriate medication use and that we are optimizing human well-being." With human factors engineering, it is possible to apply a process to the design of a system, in this case labels and labeling, to ultimately decrease the risk in that system, she explained.

Turning to the subject of the guidance FDA has issued regarding labels and labeling (CDER, 2013), Chan noted that much of this guidance was developed based on submitted reports from patients, manufacturers, and health care providers. These reports help the agency learn what is happening in the real world. She explained that FDA always encourages companies to understand their end users and the environments in which the information will be used when designing their labels and labeling. "We want sponsors to assess and obviously minimize the risk for medication errors that could be attributed to poor design of labels and labeling," said Chan.

[2] This section is based on the presentation by Irene Chan, deputy director in the Division of Medication Error Prevention and Analysis at the U.S. Food and Drug Administration, and the statements are not endorsed or verified by the National Academies of Sciences, Engineering, and Medicine.

[3] FDA defines "label" as any display of written, printed, or graphic matter on the immediate container of any article, or any such matter affixed to any consumer commodity or affixed to or appearing on a package containing any consumer commodity, and "labeling" as all written, printed, or graphic matter accompanying an article at any time while such article is in interstate commerce or held for sale after shipment or delivery in interstate commerce.

"Then we encourage the use of human factors engineering processes and gathering data through human factors studies to help characterize the risk and develop risk mitigation strategies." Human factors studies are generally smaller and quicker to complete than clinical studies, and for a small investment of resources, human factors studies can avoid the need to resolve issues postmarketing, she said.

In many cases, said Chan, designing for the user means designing for multiple end users. A product might be used by a 5-year-old and a 65-year-old, for example. "We have to understand all of the differences in the distinct patient populations and how they are going to impact how we design the products and their labels and labeling," said Chan. Understanding the user means considering if users will have vision, hearing, or tactile sense impairments, or are challenged in terms of strength and dexterity. Users may have comorbidities, low health literacy, and differences in their ability and willingness to learn. They may use the drugs in different environments. All of these factors can affect how a user is going to interact with the labels, the labeling, and the packaging and how well they can comprehend the information put before them.

In February 2016, FDA published a draft guidance on human factors studies for combinations products (CDER, 2016). This document refers to two stages of development and associated studies, and the principles described can be applied to label and labeling design as well. Formative studies are iterative in nature and involve rapid prototyping, testing the resulting designs for their ability to convey key information to patients, and using the findings to refine labels and labeling. Validation studies could evaluate what a company believes are the labels and labeling it wants to use for commercial products in the market. Validation studies generate the data that can support the claim that the user interfaces, including the labels and labeling, provide effective information for end users that will lead to safe and effective use of a given drug. Chan noted that labels and labeling by themselves will not replace good product design. "Trying to use labels and labeling to overcome, if you will, the weaknesses in something that may have been poorly designed is not really the strategy that FDA is looking for companies to take," said Chan. What FDA does expect is for manufacturers to study what they intend to put into the market and what they intend to submit in their marketing application. "We expect them to be evaluating the entire user interface—the connection points where a user, such as a patient, is going to interact with that product, and it includes the product itself, the packaging, and all of the labels and labeling that go on it and accompany it," said Chan. FDA also expects companies to evaluate products on representative users in representative scenarios with the goal of observing where there may be errors and understand why those errors are occurring.

Manufacturers use another type of study, the knowledge task study, when FDA wants to know that labels and labeling convey certain critical information correctly. "There are some things that you cannot directly observe," said Chan. "I can observe whether someone can hold an injection in place, but I may not be able to observe whether they understand if they have this particular indication or contraindication or if they are actively bleeding whether they should proceed with using the product." Such studies, then, focus on the understanding and interpretation of important user interface information.

Within the Center for Drug Evaluation and Research, the Division of Medication Error Prevention Analysis is responsible for evaluating human factors data for drug product submissions. Colleagues in FDA's Office of Medical Policy also consult on labels and labeling and help ensure that instructions are readable as far as formatting and other readability factors are concerned and at the appropriate reading level. The Office of Medical Policy's patient labeling team also makes sure that the patient package inserts, medication guides, and instructions for use employ simple words and concepts to help with patient comprehension and to ensure that unnecessary or redundant information is removed.

Going forward, said Chan, FDA is committed to the development of a new form of patient information, called Patient Medication Information, to help ensure patients receive essential information about prescription medications. FDA is proposing to amend medication guide regulations[4] to require this new form of patient labeling, which fulfill the following:

- Provide clear, concise written patient prescription drug product information.
- Be required for human prescription drug products used, dispensed, and administered on an outpatient basis.
- Have a standardized format.
- Be submitted to FDA for review and approval.
- Be distributed to patients who receive prescriptions.
- Be intended for use at home, not to replace or affect professional labeling, instructions for use, or patient counseling.
- Be freely available and easily accessible to health care providers and patients.
- Be consumer tested during development.

[4] The unified agenda listing Patient Medication Information is available at https://www.reginfo.gov/public/do/eAgendaViewRule?pubId=201604&RIN=0910-AH33 (accessed December 9, 2016).

The Patient Medication Information document would be required for human prescription drug products used, dispensed, or administered on an outpatient basis. It would have a standardized format, be submitted to FDA for review and approval, and be distributed to all patients who receive prescriptions. It would not replace labeling for professionals or the instructions for use, Chan explained in closing.

HUMAN-CENTERED DESIGN[5]

Although there are many definitions of human factors or human-centered design, Israelski favors one that says it applies data on human capabilities and characteristics to the design and evaluation of systems and devices, which can include a broad array of things, including drug labels and packaging, medical devices, smartphone apps, device and drug combinations, and websites. "Anything that has a user interface where the human has to interact, get information, process it, and then act is fair game for the field of human-centered design," said Israelski. The field has existed for more than 60 years, he explained, and relies heavily on the methods of the behavioral sciences and engineering. He noted, too, that there are many synonyms for human factors or human-centered design, such as ergonomics, usability engineering, user experience design, user-centered design, cognitive ergonomics, macroergonomics, cognitive engineering, and human engineering. Regardless of what it is called, the goal is to make products efficient, safe, and easy to learn about and use.

As Chan noted, FDA requires human-centered design in certain applications, and as a result, many good products in the medical field were developed with the help of human-centered design. In Europe, companies wishing to acquire regulatory approval must follow international standards on human factors. Many U.S. companies now employ human factors professionals, most who have a degree in the field, said Israelski. Some people come into this multidisciplinary field via one of the engineering disciplines, while others are psychologists who are interested in applying their expertise to real-world problems. Some of his colleagues have clinical backgrounds, while others come from communication fields. A few people in the field have certifications in human-centered design.

Among the award-winning products designed using human factors is a glucose meter that operates like a smartphone and takes advantage of the fact that many people are now familiar with finger gestures such as pinching and swiping. This device, said Israelski, illustrates the advantages

[5] This section is based on the presentation by Edmond Israelski, technical advisor on human factors and retired director of human factors at AbbVie Inc., and the statements are not endorsed or verified by the National Academies of Sciences, Engineering, and Medicine.

modern technology offers in terms of user interface design. So, too, does an infusion pump that has a large, readable touchscreen with a Windows-like interface that uses scrollbars, drop-down list boxes, radio buttons, and pop-up dialogue boxes. Not all human-centered design products are as complex as a glucose meter or infusion pump, he explained. Examples include an intravenous pole that is not only stable, but provides multiple places for mounting intravenous bags and storage space for an oxygen tank; ergonomic packaging for baby formula; and a hand-held, video-aided device for visualizing the vocal cords during intubation.

Israelski then described the core methods used in human-centered design (see Figure 3-1). The process starts with a contextual inquiry, which aims to understand who the likely users are and what their capabilities and limitations are, how the product will be used and in what type of scenarios, and in what environment the product will be used. Next, a risk analysis attempts to assess all the things that could go wrong when a product is in the hands of the user. This step aims to identify potential sources of error and understand how such errors might arise, whether it is because the product is lacking in some way or because users experience some type of failure, and it involves examining every task systematically for the possibil-

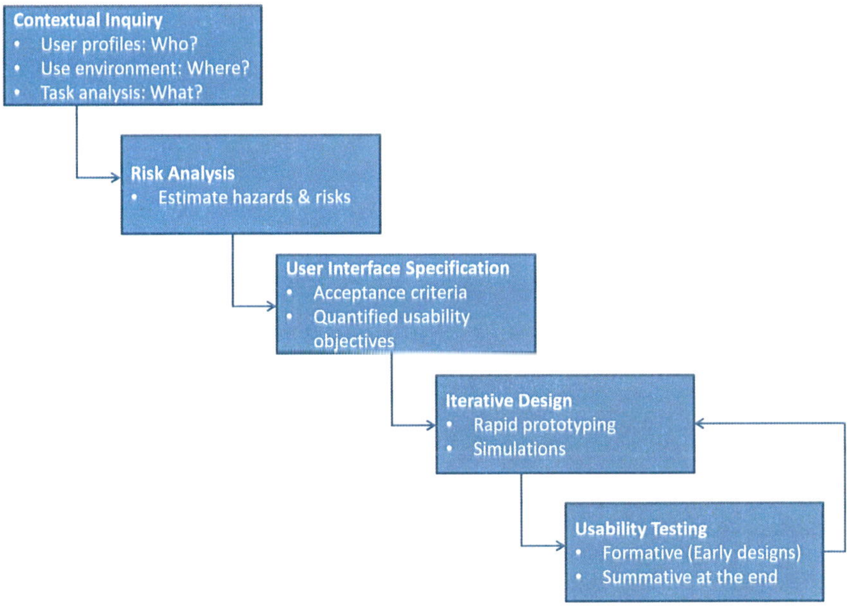

FIGURE 3-1 Human factors core methods.
SOURCE: As presented by Edmond Israelski, November 17, 2016.

ity that something could go wrong and, if so, what the consequences would be. Risk analysis helps identify the most critical and error-prone tasks that would be the leading candidates for improvement, and it is repeated after every iteration of product design.

User interface specification follows risk analysis, and it can involve working on developing user-friendly navigation features for a smartphone app or the layout of instructional materials for a medical device, for example. This step involves creating detailed specifications for user interface and product design that leaves little room for creativity on the part of the development team, according to Israelski. Assessing whether the resulting user interface does what is expected from it is usually a qualitative process when it comes to products that FDA will review, said Israelski, because a quantitative study that produces precise human factors measurements typically involves thousands of people, making them impractical and expensive.

The hard part of the human factors method, said Israelski, is the iterative and rapid prototyping and testing process. In most cases, designers conduct these early usability tests in a one-on-one environment. This setup allows the designers to observe representatives doing these tasks in a simulated environment close to the expected real-world settings in which the user would encounter the product. Following what Israelski called the initial formative iterations, the product reaches a point where it is ready to undergo validation or a summative usability test to demonstrate that all of this work has created a product that meets all of the specified user requirements and is safe and effective. He noted that while this process is not simple, it does generate products that work for all users. "We do not yet have sophisticated technology that lets you design a user interface perfectly from the beginning that will work for everybody," said Israelski. "Only through testing will you learn and iterate and make improvements." Testing does not stop once the product passes the validation process, however. "There is postmarket analysis as well in which you can learn about things that did not necessarily show up in your early work, but do show up when the product is launched. Then you can take corrective action," said Israelski.

Usability testing, he explained, is both formative and summative. Formative testing is done early with simulations and first prototypes. Its purpose is to explore user interface concepts, detect obstacles and design defects, and explore whether usability goals are attainable. This stage of testing does not necessarily have strict acceptance criteria. Summative testing, which is done in the final stage of design with the production equivalent, needs to have acceptance criteria such as usability goals for human performance and satisfaction ratings.

Addressing best practices in usability testing, Israelski said it is important to involve representative users, not just people who are convenient. If the intended users are patients with visual impairments, for example, then the five to eight people recruited for formative testing should have similar visual impairments. "We often talk about having distinct user groups," said Israelski, "and there is an art to defining them." Examples of distinct user groups, he said, would be nurses versus physicians versus patients, where each group would be assigned different tasks with different levels of risk. The test subjects are given real tasks to do, particularly critical tasks related to safety, not just convenient tasks that might make users feel good to have accomplished. "If they are not the critical tasks related to safety or the ones that are essential to getting the product used correctly or the risk communication material conveyed correctly, then you are fooling yourself by not testing the real representative task," said Israelski.

Another important step, he said, is to conduct testing in a realistic-use environment with regard to lighting, noise, and workflow. If possible, testing should use three-dimensional printed parts when testing physical products or computer simulations for products that are screen based.

Another hallmark of usability testing is asking users to think aloud and record what they do and say. It is possible to gain important insights when people are interacting with a product and the tester is encouraging the test subjects to explain what is confusing them. This "think-aloud protocol" can be helpful, Israelski said, in understanding what is going wrong in a design and where the opportunities are for making changes.

Summarizing the process, Israelski said it is systematic and scientific, and with respect to products that FDA will review, governed by rigorous design control specified by FDA. "You have to maintain a good design history file that is auditable, and you have to do formal risk management," he said. FDA requires verification to demonstrate that design outputs meet design inputs and that user interfaces meet customer requirements. The agency also requires postmarket surveillance to ensure there are no unanticipated problems.

In his final remarks, Israelski reviewed some of the human factors standards that FDA and other organizations have issued for use with medical device testing. "Even if you are not designing medical devices, they are valuable to read," said Israelski. "They tell you about the principles of human factors in some detail and how you might apply them to things like testing, risk communication, and success." He noted that these documents are long, and following them can be daunting. The American National Standards Institute/Association for the Advancement of Medical Instrumentation (ANSI/AAMI) standard HE75, for example, is 500 pages long with supplements totaling another 850 pages, but it provides valuable "getting started" information and distills 60-plus years of human factors research into actionable information. Two recently released International Electrotechnical Commission (IEC) standards, which were produced in conjunction with the International Organization for Standardization (ISO), elaborate

BOX 3-1
Human Factors Standards

- ANSI/AAMI US Domestic HF Standards [Design Principles Standard]
  - ANSI/AAMI HE 75:2009 Human factors engineering—Design of medical devices
- IEC 62366-1:2015 Medical devices—Part 1: Application of usability engineering to medical devices [Process Standard]
- IEC TR 62366-2:2016 Medical devices—Guidance on the application of usability engineering to medical devices [Process Tutorial Technical Report]

NOTE: ANSI/AAMI = American National Standards Institute/Association for the Advancement of Medical Instrumentation; IEC = International Electrotechnical Commission.
SOURCE: As presented by Edmond Israelski, November 17, 2016.

on the human factors core methods Israelski described earlier and contain tutorials for all of the methods of human factors (see Box 3-1). FDA, said Israelski, recognizes all of these standards and was heavily involved in writing them. In addition, as Chan discussed, FDA has issued several guidance documents, including one released in February 2016 that elaborates on FDA's expectations for applying human factors to medical devices.

DISCUSSION

Bernard Rosof opened the discussion by asking the panelists if human-centered design will differentiate a product in the marketplace with the economic buyer and if there are metrics to determine that. One metric, said Israelski, is whether the product succeeds in the marketplace, that people like it, adopt it, and it helps them. Diabetic patients, for example, will gravitate to glucose meters that are easier to use, less confusing, have displays that are clear and easy to read, and that track more complex factors such as meal marking and exercise. Another metric is compliance—does a product or piece of information help patients comply with their medication plans or comply with usage of a medical device? Products that improve compliance will create health, economic, and outcomes metrics that demonstrate the value of a product and that can be compared across products. Chan agreed that the marketplace is the ultimate judge of whether a product is well designed. Ultimately, she said, products that create problems such as medication errors will influence patients' willingness to use them and to recommend them to fellow consumers. She also noted that companies are starting to conduct likability testing as a means of differentiating their products, and she expects to see more of this as sponsors become more interested in how likability can affect labeling claims.

Jay Duhig from AbbVie Inc. commented that the speakers in the first panel session stated clearly that patients needed to be included more in the resource development and tool development process and that the second panel described a very systematic method for doing so, collecting data, and then creating user-centered tools in an iterative process. He noted that both Israelski and Chan had influenced a wide range of groups that are creating materials and asked if they had any thoughts on how to get organizations to increase their inclusion of patients when they develop resources. He also asked them for ideas on how to get organizations to adopt practices that reflect the research on human factors, health literacy, and usability. Israelski suggested publicizing case studies in which human-centered design has been applied successfully to develop materials that patients, physicians, health care providers, and payers find useful, particularly if they are accompanied by business cases. He said that good human-centered design that can improve patient compliance is better for patients and for payers. Demonstrating benefits from the perspective of patients and health economics is one way of getting these methods adopted more widely, he said. Chan agreed that getting consumers more involved in the design of medication materials is a key aspect of getting patient-centered design widely adopted.

Israelski recommended a book, *Cost Justifying Usability*, by Randolph Bias and Deborah Mayhew, that presents business cases showing how human factors can produce an economic return to the companies employing its methods. As an example, he said that many medical products suffer recalls or returns that are tied to usability issues. "If you can show in a little business case that you have put a dent in that rate—say it was originally 10 percent and now you bring it down to 5 percent—you can put a dollar value onto that increase in customer acceptance and decrease in complaints." Compared to the outlay for human factors, which is typically small compared to that of clinical trials, the return on investment will be high, said Israelski.

He also pointed to the importance of regulatory power. For example, before the human factors group moved to the FDA Office of Device Evaluation, it was simply a consulting group that was not required to be involved in every review. They are involved in the review process today, and the result, he said, has been "amazing" in that companies are now creating human factors groups. "This is all due to FDA," said Israelski, who added that big pharmaceuticals did not have human factors groups before this change at FDA. "This has been a great boon for people in human factors as a profession," said Israelski.

Ruth Parker said that Chan's remarks about FDA's emphasis on health literacy and involving patients and payers was "music to my ears" and an important sign of progress. She then asked Shrank to comment on what happens to products designed using human factors once they reach the market and how health literacy plays out in the postapproval world. Shrank replied that postmarket surveillance research today is generally epidemiologic in nature and leverages large databases. "It looks at rates of clinical outcomes by patients depending on what meds they are taking and what combination of meds they are taking, but there is little nuance around the patient's experience of how they take their meds," said Shrank. As to why some medications work better than others in the real world, he said there are biologic and genetic reasons, social reasons beyond adherence, the way in which drugs are administered, and the ways in which patients manage their lifestyles. "I think the concept of a much richer, patient-centered view of data collection could allow for a much richer and more nuanced way of understanding more about safety, efficacy, and adherence in the postmarketing surveillance time period," said Shrank. "I do hope that is something that could be expanded on."

Chan, speaking from FDA's perspective, said the Center for Drug Evaluation and Research uses the FDA Adverse Event Reporting System, which receives millions of reports from manufacturers, as a major data source. It also relies on reports consumers and providers submit directly to the agency and from patient safety organizations such as the Institute for Safe Medication Practices. Each of these data sources is important and scrutinized by FDA, said Chan, for they identify where patients and providers are finding difficulty understanding medication information. She believes the marketplace provides the only true test of how understandable medication materials are. "Whatever the manufacturers do in terms of simulated testing before they bring something to market is not going to compare to getting it into the hands of potentially millions of users and then seeing what gets reported to the agency," said Chan. "Postmarketing is very important for the agency and something we pay attention to in driving policy recommendations," she said.

Israelski commented on the rise of social media and said both patients and members of the health care system are gleaning a great deal of postmarket information from Facebook and Twitter as well as websites devoted to specific diseases. "People readily tell their stories," he said. "On YouTube, you can find people teaching you how to deal with side effects and the risks of certain medications and therapies with a great amount of detail." In his opinion, these social media outlets and websites create an opportunity for patients and families to learn about various health conditions and to educate themselves about the pros and cons of different therapies and alternatives so they can ask intelligent questions of their doctors before making health care decisions. "There is the downside of too much information and some of it being bad, but I think on the balance, what we have available to us is a wonderful thing. I think it makes postmarket surveillance even richer because of that," said Israelski.

An unidentified workshop participant asked the panelists for examples of approaches that have worked, and Shrank provided several examples of how CVS used human factors to develop a variety of approaches on how patients administer their medications. One approach synchronizes all of a patient's prescription refills on the same day of the month so they do not have to make multiple trips to the pharmacy. Another tactic creates multidose packs containing all of a patient's morning doses in one pack and their evening doses in another pack. "This is a much simpler way to administer a complex drug regimen," said Shrank. CVS has also created a series of incentives to encourage people to engage in healthy behaviors, including one in which they leveraged behavioral economics to get people to stop smoking (Halpern et al., 2015).

Israelski noted that AbbVie has had a number of successes using human factors in its product designs. For the biologic drug Humira, which has been approved to treat a number of autoimmune diseases, AbbVie created supportive apps for patients and a talking training pen and video to teach patients how to inject the drug properly. These tools have worked well enough that there is a very low rate of patients not being able to use the injector successfully, which is a big part of compliance. The company used human factors to design packaging and labeling for hepatitis C drugs and for complicated regimens of oral oncology drugs. "The packaging and labeling designs have to be done right to get those schedules understood and used properly by patients to get the drug to be used safely and effectively," said Israelski. Human factors helped AbbVie design an ambulatory infusion pump for Parkinson's disease that individuals with impairment caused by tremor and stiffness can use. "The company has embraced human factors and seen the pay-off," he added.

Elisabeth Walther from the Office of Medical Policy at FDA responded to a question about a proposed rule change that would require a one-page patient-centered medication information sheet to accompany all drugs dispensed or administered on an outpatient basis. She noted that this rule change has been included on the spring 2017 Unified Agenda, which lists the regulations FDA expects to publish within the next year. Chan added that the industry now realizes that ensuring patients know how to use a drug is part of FDA's consideration as to whether a product is safe and effective. "That has been a message that we have been trying to drive home to our stakeholders," said Chan.

Rosof noted that the issue of medication safety and health literacy was first raised in 2000 and 2001 with the release of two Institute of Medicine reports, *To Err Is Human* (IOM, 2000) and *Crossing the Quality Chasm* (IOM, 2001). These two reports described quality as a systems property, yet he has not heard a discussion about these issues within integrated delivery systems, including his own. "What are we missing here in terms of translating this discussion to where medication use is a real issue?" asked Rosof. Shrank replied that there is a clearer sense of what needs to be done in the somewhat controlled environment of a hospital and there has been an extraordinary effort and success with regard to medication safety in that environment. Doing the same thing with patients in their homes is more difficult, he said, in part because "the patient may not always be aligned in terms of what their perceptions are of success. Patients have varying views about the value of their medication and how they feel about their medication. If the patient at any point is not aligned, that is going to be a very hard thing to overcome," said Shrank.

Another contributor to this challenge, he said, is that so many social factors affect a patient's decision about how to take their medications at home, making it difficult to create a systematic approach that addresses them all. "Things such as the cultural features of taking medication, the cost of taking medication, the unexpected fact that your car broke down and you cannot get to the pharmacy, or your arthritis is acting up and you cannot open the bottle" were factors that Shrank described. "The number of permutations of potential barriers is almost infinite." The answer, he added, is to keep creating better systems, such as multidose packaging, and engaging in efforts to help support, engage, and motivate patients. He acknowledged, though, that the weakest point in the system is when patients are discharged, particularly when patients have to reconcile the medications they receive at discharge with the medications they have at home. UPMC pharmacists now do a face-to-face medication reconciliation with patients at discharge, which Shrank said is having a positive impact on compliance and safety.

Rosof then asked Chan if FDA was satisfied with how health systems are performing in this regard. She replied that safety issues in a health care system do not fall under FDA's purview. She added, however, that her division at FDA thinks a great deal about the entire medication use system. "We think about how that product is traveling through all of the different settings of care and whose hands are on it and who is interacting with it when we think about how we want to make recommendations or what recommendations we want to take," she explained. Historically, she noted, the agency took a reactive approach, where it would react to a postmarketing issue, but today the agency is more proactive at identifying points in the medication use system that are vulnerable to failure. "We expect that manufacturers are going out there and really understanding their users in their home environments and their settings of care to design a better product," said Chan. She believes that while some of that work aims to meet FDA requirements, companies are intentional about designing a product that can be used safely and effectively in the hands of its customers. "I think it is important to underscore that that kind of research can be done early in development by manufacturers," Chan added.

Daniel Morrow from the University of Illinois commented that while he had heard about the potential of technology for integration and improving the patient experience and the crucial role of human factors in realizing that potential, he has not heard anyone discuss the potential for the electronic health record (EHR) to be the lynchpin of the synergy between the health care system and the home. He asked if FDA is playing a role in promoting the use of EHRs to support self-care in coordination with their providers. Walther replied that FDA has in fact considered that issue when it developed the proposed new Patient Medication Information rule and has included flexibility in the rule that should enable EHR vendors to develop applications that could support better communication between the health care system and the patient at home.

Israelski commented that a company such as AbbVie has to embrace the entire health care ecosystem and how its products fit into the patient journey. "We have meetings where we look at the patient journey from diagnosis to original prescription to titration, maintenance, and hopefully, cure or stable conditions," he said. This mapping exercise enables the company to identify the things it can develop, such as training materials, doctors' aids, and other types of information, to help enhance the patient journey through the health care ecosystem. One question AbbVie is asking, he added, is how supportive features such as apps and websites integrate with the EHR to improve the patient journey.

Shrank noted that UPMC has a care management tool that integrates with the EHR. Care managers, nurse practitioners, allied staff, and pharmacists use this tool to manage patients and coordinate their care over time. "For us, it is not an EHR thing. It is finding the right place within the workflow that delivers the right information to the person that is going to do the outreach," he explained.

Darvece Monson remarked that she appreciated both the opportunity to hear from those who are working on these problems and how difficult these challenges are to address. She then said that simplicity is what empowers patients, and therefore simplicity is the most important factor to remember when designing products. As an example, a warning that a drug may cause a decrease in blood pressure could be accompanied by a link to a webpage that explains exactly what that means and describes the signs of a decrease in blood pressure. "Something as simple as that can help the patient become more empowered and involved in their care," said Monson.

Walther ended the discussion by stating that FDA values anytime patients can provide the agency with information on what they need. "It really does influence what we do," said Walther. She encouraged patients to contact FDA with their concerns at patientmedicationinformation@fda.gov.

4

Translating Research into Practice: Case Studies

The workshop's third panel session featured four case studies illustrating how health systems are translating research into practice. Steve Sparks, health literacy director for Wisconsin Health Literacy, described a statewide effort in Wisconsin to adopt health-literate medication labels, and Laurie Myers, global health literacy director at Merck Sharp & Dohme Corp., discussed the importance of including individuals with low health literacy in efforts to develop new medication labeling for patients. Brian Jack, professor and chair of the Department of Family Medicine at the Boston University School of Medicine, reviewed Project RED, an effort to reduce rehospitalization using a redesigned discharge process, and Charles Lee, president and founder of Polyglot Systems, spoke about approaches for providing medication information to non-English speakers. Following the four presentations, Donna Horn, director of patient safety–community pharmacy at the Institute for Safe Medication Practices, and H. Shonna Yin, associate professor of pediatrics and population health in the Departments of Pediatrics and Population Health at the New York University School of Medicine and Bellevue Hospital Center, gave their reactions to the four presentations. An open discussion moderated by Bernard Rosof followed the comments from the reactors.

ADOPTING AN EASY-TO-READ MEDICATION LABEL IN WISCONSIN[1]

As an introduction to his presentation on Wisconsin Health Literacy's efforts to improve medication labels in Wisconsin, Steve Sparks noted that whenever he talks about this work, he hears stories about how medication errors have led to near disasters. "The stories we hear serve as a constant reminder of just how important our work really is," said Sparks. His work, he explained, began shortly after U.S. Pharmacopeia (USP) issued new patient-centered labeling guidelines in 2013. The Wisconsin Partnership Program of the University of Wisconsin School of Medicine and Public Health provided funding for this work.

Phase 1 of this project involved interviewing pharmacists and pharmacy managers working at both independent and chain pharmacies, as well as representatives from companies that provide software used to generate labels in those pharmacies. He and his colleagues also interviewed physicians and stakeholders from states that had already implemented patient-centered guidelines. These interviews revealed that most pharmacists were not aware of the new guidelines or had forgotten USP had issued them. However, once the new guidelines were explained, pharmacists supported them, believed they would improve readability and reduce confusion, and believed they did not need additional evidence to convince them to adopt the new label given the clear benefits of doing so. The pharmacists also thought the guidelines were compatible with current pharmacy workflows, though they were concerned about the limited space on labels and the flexibility of pharmacy software programs to produce labels meeting the new guidelines. Other potential barriers pharmacists mentioned included organizational acceptance and the cost of buying new label stock. The pharmacists mentioned that many customers request the medication's purpose on their labels, but explained that most pharmacies do not have access to that information. The interviews with stakeholders found that while some states have patient-centered label standards in place, only one state had tried to mandate the USP standards, and this effort was not as successful as anticipated.

Energized by the findings of the first phase of this project, Wisconsin Health Literacy applied for and received a grant from the Medical College of Wisconsin's Advancing a Healthier Wisconsin Endowment to pilot redesigned labels in 52 pharmacies in the southern and eastern parts of the state. The pharmacies included those serving low-income neighborhoods, rural areas of the state, and health care systems. Together, they issue 1.8 million

[1] This section is based on the presentation by Steve Sparks, health literacy director for Wisconsin Health Literacy, and the statements are not endorsed or verified by the National Academies of Sciences, Engineering, and Medicine.

prescriptions per year, and each of the three pharmacy systems involved used a different pharmacy software: Rx30, EnterpriseRx by McKesson, and PioneerRx. "This was valuable to us because it will give us experience in expanding implementation to more pharmacies in the future and looking at how the process may be implemented or may be impacted by the individual software that they are using," explained Sparks. The goal of phase 2 of this project is to implement and evaluate the USP guidelines by redesigning labels in the pilot pharmacies by the end of 2017 and use the experience gained in this pilot phase to more efficiently and smoothly implement the standards statewide in the project's third phase. He noted that based on earlier research and the experience of other states, Wisconsin Health Literacy will pursue a voluntary adoption strategy rather than a mandatory one.

As part of the phase 2 pilots, which began on January 1, 2016, Wisconsin Health Literacy established a project advisory committee that included pharmacy partners, health literacy experts such as Michael Wolf, and representatives from USP, the Pharmacy Society of Wisconsin, and Epic, the electronic health record (EHR) vendor that happens to be located in Madison, Wisconsin. Phase 2 also included patient focus groups made up of individuals who Sparks described as those who "typically may not have had a voice in a project such as this but whose input is essential for the work that we're doing." The focus groups, he explained, were helpful in determining what information should be included where on the label. He noted, too, that one of the most interesting activities had the focus groups design their own labels (see Figure 4-1).

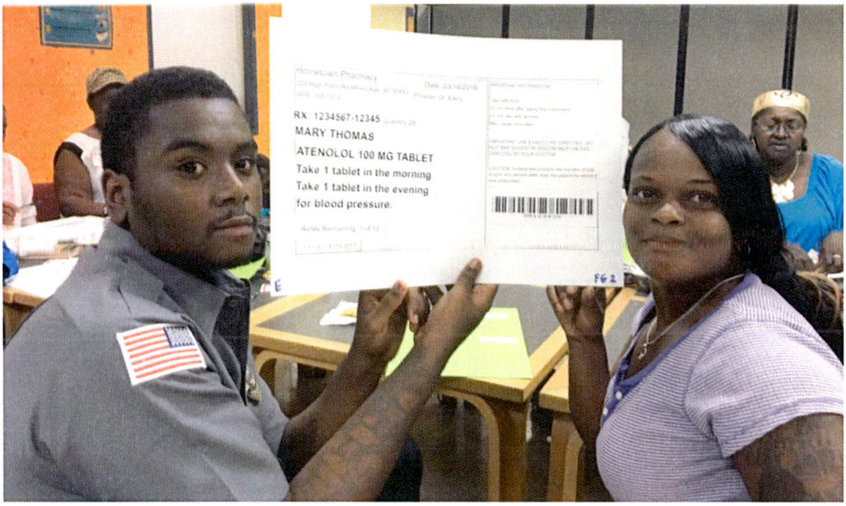

FIGURE 4-1 A prescription label designed by focus group members.
SOURCE: As presented by Steve Sparks, November 17, 2016.

One benefit of involving focus groups, said Sparks, is that the enthusiastic members were willing to share their stories about medication issues. "One woman told us she had a terrible experience because she was taking care of her mother, who had diabetes. She had all kinds of medications that she was giving to her mother, was so confused about the instructions, and was just afraid she would do something that would be disastrous to her mother and her mother's health." Other comments, though not directly applicable to the project, said Sparks, were thought provoking. For example, some focus group members believed pharmacies are here to help, but others held the strong opinion that pharmacies just want to make money. "And another observation, perhaps the most interesting," he said, "was the perception that pharmacies give lower quality medication to the poor." A number of people in the focus groups, he added, believed that generic drugs were given to the poor.

Sparks and his collaborators also started a patient advisory council made up of community members, one of whom is also on the project advisory council. The patient group meets quarterly and examines and comments on surveys and other communications. By working with these different groups, his team has produced several labels, still in the working-draft phase (see Figure 4-2), that pilot pharmacies will use starting in December 2016.

On April 3, 2017, Sparks and his team members will hold a day-long medication label summit featuring testimonials from the participating pharmacy members, as well as presentations by health literacy experts such as Wolf and Ruth Parker. This event, said Sparks, will serve as a key opportunity to share learnings and encourage other pharmacies to adopt the new labels in phase 3. One lesson learned so far is that each pharmacy has its own process and a unique relationship with the software vendor. "You cannot work with a pharmacy without working directly with the software vendor," he explained.

A second lesson is that every pharmacy differs in how it wants to adopt new labels. Some, said Sparks, are willing to throw out all of the old label stock and start from scratch. Others have tens of thousands of labels in a storeroom that they want to use, which leads to work-arounds that can apply new standards to old color blocks and logo placement. Some pharmacies, he noted, insist on including information not in the USP guidelines and not required by law, but important to their workflow. One pharmacy, for example, wants to include the National Drug Code number—a unique 10-digit number that identifies the labeler, product, and trade package size—on the label, and several want to include the medication description. "While still adhering to the USP standards, we were able to be flexible and accommodate these requests," said Sparks.

One important lesson is that pharmacy team involvement in label redesign and implementation is critical for success. "It was important the

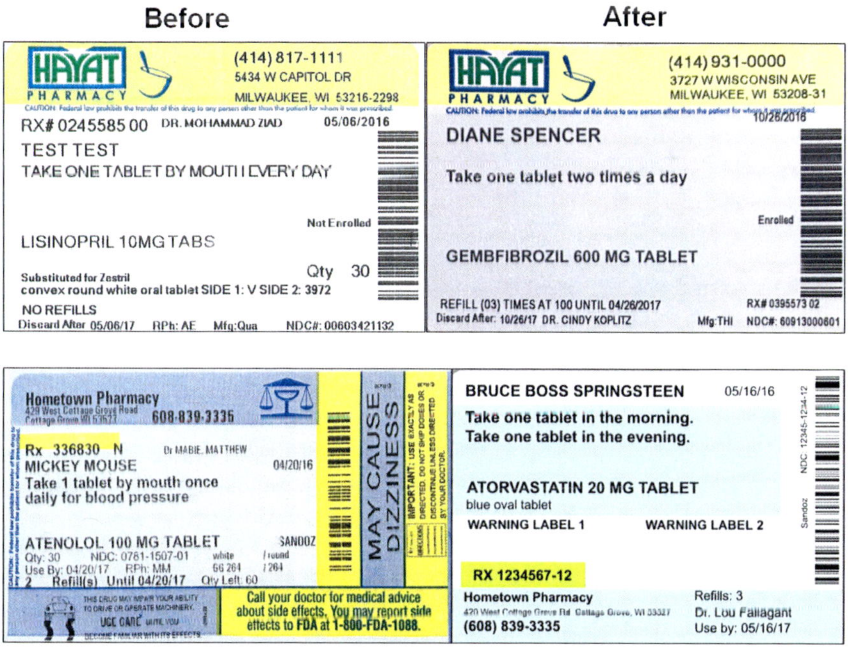

FIGURE 4-2 Current and working-draft redesigned labels.
SOURCE: As presented by Steve Sparks, November 17, 2016.

pharmacies felt we were working with them to come up with the new labels and the processes, not just giving them a set of standards they had to adopt," said Sparks. "I do not think that would have worked, and as a result, the process is going much smoother and faster." In the same vein, involving major stakeholders, including pharmacy boards and major pharmacy chains, makes for a smoother adoption process. Representatives from major pharmacy chains, he said, have been largely positive about this project while acknowledging the challenges of working across multiple sites.

Several issues also arose during the label design process that will require further study, largely related to the complexity of resolving those issues and the outside systems that would have to change as a result. The example Sparks cited was that adding the medication purpose on the label will require a massive change by providers and in the EHR software. Another issue involves how to standardize medication dosage instructions, for which there are no universally accepted standards.

In closing, Sparks said the next steps in this project will be to work closely with the partners to monitor implementation. "We are going to be surveying patients in three pharmacy systems to see if they notice a change and if they like the new labels." One of the three systems, he said, is a Medicaid health plan serving one of the pharmacy systems, providing the opportunity to analyze medication use before and after the new labels. "We look forward to learning more and applying the information to broader interpretation and implementation of patient-centered labels across the state in the third and final phase of the project, which we hope will start in 2018," said Sparks. "We believe that the journey to better medication labels has begun and that the project could have implications well beyond the borders of Wisconsin."

INCLUDING INDIVIDUALS WITH LOW HEALTH LITERACY IN THE DEVELOPMENT AND TESTING OF PATIENT LABELING[2]

Laurie Myers, who has led Merck's health literacy work for the past 6 years, discussed how she and her colleagues included individuals with low health literacy in their work in developing and testing health-literate patient labeling for new molecules. Summarizing the key message of her presentation, Myers said, "It is important to include respondents with low health literacy. It will not happen by accident. You have to be thoughtful and make sure you do it in a systematic way, but it will give you a product that is much, much better."

The overall goal of this project, she explained, has been to maximize comprehension of patient labeling for all audiences. "We knew we wanted to do this a number of years ago, but we were not quite sure how," she said. One lesson she has learned is that it takes the involvement of multiple stakeholders to make this kind of change, including, for example, the company's attorneys who believed it was possible both to be clear to patients and to follow the letter and spirit of the law. Another lesson is that the project had to start somewhere, so she and her team began with new drugs the company was developing. "This is not about looking backward, this is about looking ahead and proactively developing health-literate labeling for new molecules," Myers explained.

What she and her colleagues realized was that while Merck has always been committed to clear patient labeling, and had previously included individuals with a broad range of education levels in its labeling design efforts, that research included few individuals with limited health literacy. Most of the people volunteering for Internet-based research on patient labels had adequate health literacy, so she and her team had to put

[2] This section is based on the presentation by Laurie Myers, global health literacy director at Merck Sharp & Dohme Corp., and the statements are not endorsed or verified by the National Academies of Sciences, Engineering, and Medicine.

into place different health literacy assessments to ensure they had enough people with low health literacy on their test panels to make a systematic assessment of how well panel members understood the information on patient labeling.

Merck's revamped process for developing and testing patient labeling for new drugs starts with creating draft labeling that is accurate and consistent with physician labeling. Health literacy experts, including Parker, Wolf, and their teams, then review the draft labeling and suggest changes based on best practices in health literacy. After Merck reviews and approves the suggested changes, Parker, Wolf, and their teams conduct focus groups in Chicago and Atlanta that not only review the labeling for readability and clarity, but also help develop descriptions for concepts that the team is not sure how to explain in common language. For example, the focus groups might suggest words that could be used to describe a specific type of skin rash based on a picture. The company also conducts qualitative research with limited and adequate health literacy respondents to ensure the revised labeling is well understood across a range of health literacy levels. This iterative process of redesign and retesting reflects the importance of listening and responding to patients and caregivers.

To recruit individuals with low health literacy, the agency that conducts the qualitative research (Sommer Consulting) goes to places such as literacy centers and senior centers. They also included patients over age 70, as appropriate, who historically may have been excluded from such studies. Myers noted that in one recent comprehension study, two-thirds of the participants were over age 65. This change in recruiting processes illustrates the importance of questioning assumptions, said Myers. The recruitment process also includes a one-question health literacy screen in which potential respondents are asked how confident they are at filling out medical forms by themselves. This is done to make sure that there is adequate representation of participants with low health literacy. At the end of the comprehension testing, participants are also given the Newest Vital Sign (NVS) assessment, the results of which Myers and her team use for a final classification of the health literacy level of the panel members. "When you think about managing your health and managing your disease, numeracy is such an important part of that, and the NVS gets at that better," she explained. She noted that Schlesinger Associates, which many companies in the pharmaceutical industry use for market research recruitment, is now adding the one-question health literacy screen to the profiles of potential participants in its subject database.

The recruitment goal for comprehension testing is to have 25 percent of the participants be individuals with low health literacy. "Sometimes we do not get there, but we usually come close," said Myers. She added that the risk factors for chronic disease are often the same as the risk factors for low health literacy, further pointing to the importance of including individuals with low health literacy in labeling assessments.

Today, the qualitative research (comprehension testing) is conducted both in-person and online. It is easier to recruit respondents with low health literacy to in-person market research. An important part of this effort, she explained, is to work with a market research company that is sensitized to the principles of health literacy and to treating low health-literacy individuals, who may not always be confident talking about medical information, with respect and dignity. "These are the kinds of soft things that make this successful," said Myers. Her team now does both open- and closed-book assessments. Closed-book assessments provide insights into whether people, without being able to look at anything, can say, "What is it for? How do you take it? What are the serious side effects? What are the common side effects?" she explained. However, in the real world today, people go online when they have a question about a medication, making it important to include open-book testing as well.

Another change to Merck's assessment procedure is that it no longer includes the requirement that people have a computer to participate in comprehension testing. "We used to require a desktop computer, but many people of lower socioeconomic status are more likely to have a phone, not a desktop, to access the Internet," explained Myers. This inadvertently excluded those people from qualitative research, she added. The company also starts the recruitment process earlier than it used to because it takes more time to identify individuals with low health literacy.

Myers presented the overall results of multiple rounds of qualitative research testing patient labeling. The results showed there was high comprehension by respondents with both adequate and limited health literacy. Today, when Merck submits its patient labeling for new molecules, the company provides a brief summary of the results of this research to the U.S. Food and Drug Administration (FDA) to demonstrate that the company has evidence the label is well understood.

While in general it is true that people with less education have lower levels of health literacy and that those with more education have higher levels of health literacy, education is not a perfect proxy for health literacy. "The amazing thing is, people with more education are more likely to have higher comprehension, but even people with even only some high school are able to understand [the patient labeling developed from] this process," said Myers. The same is true of age, where comprehension among older adults may be a little less, she said, but even people who are older are able to understand the new patient labels.

Not surprisingly, said Myers, patients love the new draft patient labeling. In follow-up interviews, participants say that health-literate labeling would make it likely they would read the information, keep the informa-

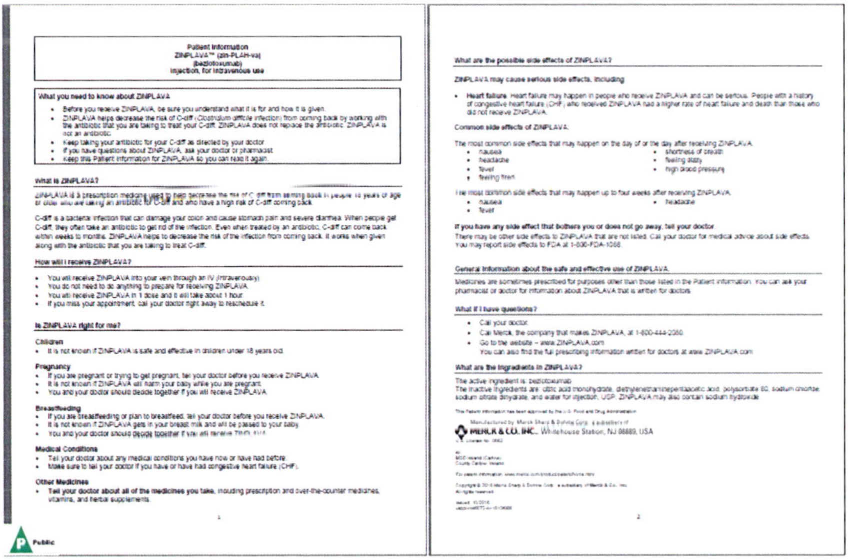

Patient Information
ZINPLAVA™ (zin-PLAH-va)
(bezlotoxumab)
injection, for intravenous use

What you need to know about ZINPLAVA

- Before you receive ZINPLAVA, be sure you understand what it is for and how it is given.
- ZINPLAVA helps decrease the risk of C-diff (Clostridium difficile infection) from coming back by working with the antibiotic that you are taking to treat your C-diff. ZINPLAVA does not replace the antibiotic. ZINPLAVA is not an antibiotic.
- Keep taking your antibiotic for your C-diff as directed by your doctor.
- If you have questions about ZINPLAVA, ask your doctor or pharmacist.
- Keep this Patient Information for ZINPLAVA so you can read it again.

What is ZINPLAVA?

ZINPLAVA is a prescription medicine used to help decrease the risk of C-diff from coming back in people 18 years of age or older who are taking an antibiotic for C-diff and who have a high risk of C-diff coming back.

C-diff is a bacterial infection that can damage your colon and cause stomach pain and severe diarrhea. When people get C-diff, they often take an antibiotic to get rid of the infection. Even when treated by an antibiotic, C-diff can come back within weeks to months. ZINPLAVA helps to decrease the risk of the infection from coming back. It works when given along with the antibiotic that you are taking to treat C-diff.

How will I receive ZINPLAVA?

- You will receive ZINPLAVA into your vein through an IV (intravenously).
- You do not need to do anything to prepare for receiving ZINPLAVA.
- You will receive ZINPLAVA in 1 dose and it will take about 1 hour.
- If you miss your appointment, call your doctor right away to reschedule it.

Is ZINPLAVA right for me?

Children
- It is not known if ZINPLAVA is safe and effective in children under 18 years old.

Pregnancy
- If you are pregnant or trying to get pregnant, tell your doctor before you receive ZINPLAVA.
- It is not known if ZINPLAVA will harm your baby while you are pregnant.
- You and your doctor should decide together if you will receive ZINPLAVA.

Breastfeeding
- If you are breastfeeding or plan to breastfeed, tell your doctor before you receive ZINPLAVA.
- It is not known if ZINPLAVA gets in your breast milk and will be passed to your baby.
- You and your doctor should decide together if you will receive ZINPLAVA.

Medical Conditions
- Tell your doctor about any medical conditions you have now or have had before.
- Make sure to tell your doctor if you have or have had congestive heart failure (CHF).

Other Medicines
- **Tell your doctor about all of the medicines you take,** including prescription and over-the-counter medicines, vitamins, and herbal supplements.

1

Public

What are the possible side effects of ZINPLAVA?

ZINPLAVA may cause serious side effects, including:

- **Heart failure.** Heart failure may happen in people who receive ZINPLAVA and can be serious. People with a history of congestive heart failure (CHF) who received ZINPLAVA had a higher rate of heart failure and death than those who did not receive ZINPLAVA.

Common side effects of ZINPLAVA:

The most common side effects that may happen on the day of or the day after receiving ZINPLAVA:
- nausea
- headache
- fever
- feeling tired
- shortness of breath
- feeling dizzy
- high blood pressure

The most common side effects that may happen up to four weeks after receiving ZINPLAVA:
- nausea
- fever
- headache

If you have any side effect that bothers you or does not go away, tell your doctor.
There may be other side effects to ZINPLAVA that are not listed. Call your doctor for medical advice about side effects. You may report side effects to FDA at 1-800-FDA-1088.

General information about the safe and effective use of ZINPLAVA.

Medicines are sometimes prescribed for purposes other than those listed in the Patient Information. You can ask your pharmacist or doctor for information about ZINPLAVA that is written for doctors.

What if I have questions?

- Call your doctor.
- Call Merck, the company that makes ZINPLAVA, at 1-800-444-2080.
- Go to the website – www.ZINPLAVA.com
  You can also find the full prescribing information written for doctors at www.ZINPLAVA.com

What are the ingredients in ZINPLAVA?

The active ingredient is: bezlotoxumab
The inactive ingredients are: citric acid monohydrate, diethylenetriaminepentaacetic acid, polysorbate 80, sodium chloride, sodium citrate dihydrate, and water for injection, USP. ZINPLAVA may also contain sodium hydroxide.

Manufactured by: Merck Sharp & Dohme Corp., a subsidiary of
MERCK & CO., INC., Whitehouse Station, NJ 08889, USA

2

FIGURE 4-3 Patient labeling created through Merck's new process to create health-literate labeling.
SOURCES: As presented by Laurie Myers, November 17, 2016.

tion as a reference, have a clear understanding of how to use a medication correctly and the risks involved, and be able to ask questions of their providers. One request that participants have made is for labeling to include information about the risks and benefits of their medicines, though Myers acknowledged that type of information is not something that is likely to be included in the near future.

As an example of labeling created through this process, Myers showed the FDA-approved labeling for ZINPLAVA[3] (see Figure 4-3). She gave FDA kudos for supporting Merck's efforts to apply health literacy principles to the development of its patient labeling.

In a new project, Myers and her team, in partnership with Wolf, Parker, and their colleagues, are using a similar process to develop and test the Instructions for Use document. "The long and short of it is, this is working well and much like with patient labeling, we have to have an open mind,"

---

[3] For full prescribing information, or any future labeling updates, please see the physician and patient labeling available at www.zinplava.com.

she said. For example, in the first prototype developed, instructions used to say "swirl for 30 to 60 seconds," which meant the patient had to have a watch or use their phone. Instead, instructions now say "count to 45," which she said is much easier than having to use a clock. "Little things like that that just are really about thinking differently and thinking innovatively," said Myers. The initial results of testing these new instructions have been positive. Based on early results and testing, even people with limited health literacy have had more success in measuring and mixing medicines safely, she said.

In closing, Myers said that just because this process works in patient labeling does not mean it will work automatically in other types of consumer research without careful thought. "You have to think about this one project at a time," she said. "It is possible, though, to develop information about new products that is simple and clear and easily understood by people of all health literacy levels."

PROJECT RED: ENGAGING PATIENTS IN MEDICATION MANAGEMENT AT HOSPITAL DISCHARGE[4]

Brian Jack began his presentation by listing the 11 mutually reinforcing components (see Box 4-1) of the Reengineered Discharge Program (Project RED) that he and his colleagues developed with the assistance of the Agency for Healthcare Research and Quality (AHRQ) (Jack et al., 2008; Mitchell et al., 2010, 2012). Medication reconciliation sits at the top of this list because it is the most important component of a health-literate discharge program, said Jack. Other critical components, he added, are the written discharge plan—a health-literate document that patients and their caregivers can use at home—and an assessment of patient understanding using techniques such as teach-back and a follow-up telephone call, again to measure understanding and to answer questions. He noted that the discharge plan is different from the discharge summary, which goes to the patient's primary care provider. In 2006, the National Quality Forum adopted Project RED as the standard for hospital discharge and as the 11th of 30 Safe Practices (NQF, 2006).[5]

To test the effectiveness of Project RED, Jack and his colleagues conducted a randomized, controlled trial on 749 patients who received usual care or the RED intervention (Jack et al., 2009). In the intervention, a nurse acts as the discharge educator, collecting information from clinical

[4] This section is based on the presentation by Brian Jack, professor and chair of the Department of Family Medicine at the Boston University School of Medicine, and the statements are not endorsed or verified by the National Academies of Sciences, Engineering, and Medicine.

[5] It is now the 15th of 34 Safe Practices listed in the 2010 update (NQF, 2010).

BOX 4-1
The 11 Mutually Reinforcing Components of a Health-Literate Discharge Program

1. Medication reconciliation
2. Reconcile discharge plan with national guidelines
3. Follow-up appointments
4. Outstanding tests
5. Postdischarge services
6. Written discharge plan
7. What to do if problem arises
8. Patient education
9. Assess patient understanding
10. Discharge summary to primary care provider
11. Telephone reinforcement

SOURCE: As presented by Brian Jack, November 17, 2016.

staff, packaging that information, and then teaching the patient how to use this information in their posthospitalization care. The nurse educator also reviews the formal after-hospital care plan with the patient, uses teach-back methods to ensure the patient and family members understand the plan, and relays the plan to the patient's primary care provider. A clinical pharmacist calls patients 2 to 4 days after discharge to reinforce the discharge plan and review medications. The results of the trial showed that fewer patients who received the Project RED intervention had to return to the hospital for any reason compared with patients who received the then-standard discharge process.

Focusing on the after-hospital care plan, Jack said that he and his colleagues spent a great deal of time thinking about how to create this document so that patients of all levels of health literacy would have the best chance of understanding what they needed to do after leaving the hospital. The resulting document makes liberal use of white space, large fonts, pictures, and icons (see Figure 4-4), and the medication component is structured to answer the four questions that focus groups identified as the most common that patients want answered: What time of day do I take this medicine?, Why am I taking this medication?, How much do I take?, and How do I take this medicine? (see Figure 4-5). An important aspect of the medication page, Jack noted, is what it does not contain: information about pathophysiology or mechanism of action. An evaluation of the after-

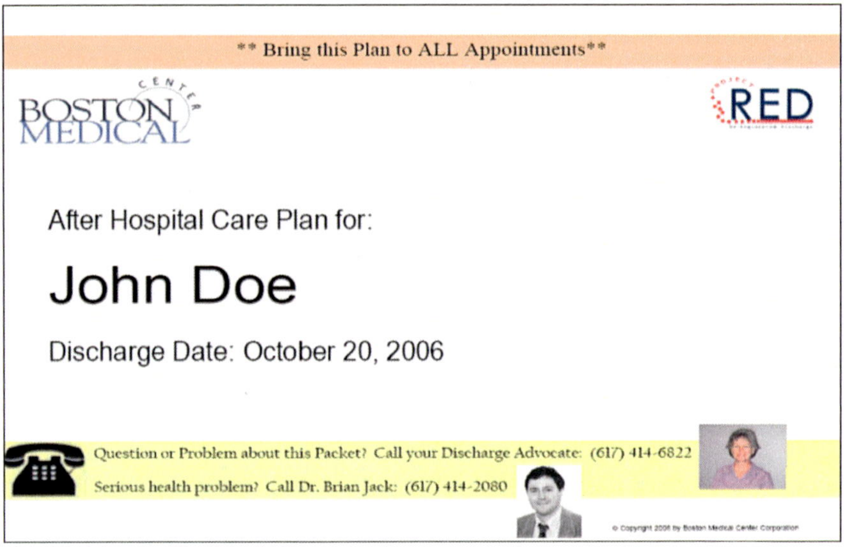

FIGURE 4-4 Personalized cover page of an after-hospital care plan.
SOURCE: As presented by Brian Jack, November 17, 2016.

EACH DAY follow this schedule:

MEDICINES

What time of day do I take this medicine?	Why am I taking this medicine?	Medication name Amount	How much do I take?	How do I take this medicine?
Morning	blood pressure	PROCARDIA XL NIFEDIPINE 90 mg	1 pill	By mouth
	blood pressure	HYDROCHLOROTHIAZIDE 25 mg	1 pill	By mouth
	blood pressure	CLONIDINE HCl 0.1 mg	3 pills	By mouth
	cholesterol	LIPITOR ATORVASTATIN CALCIUM 20 mg	1 pill	By mouth
	stomach	PROTONIX PANTOPRAZOLE SODIUM 40 mg	1 pill	By mouth

FIGURE 4-5 Medication instructions in an after-hospital care plan.
SOURCE: As presented by Brian Jack, November 17, 2016.

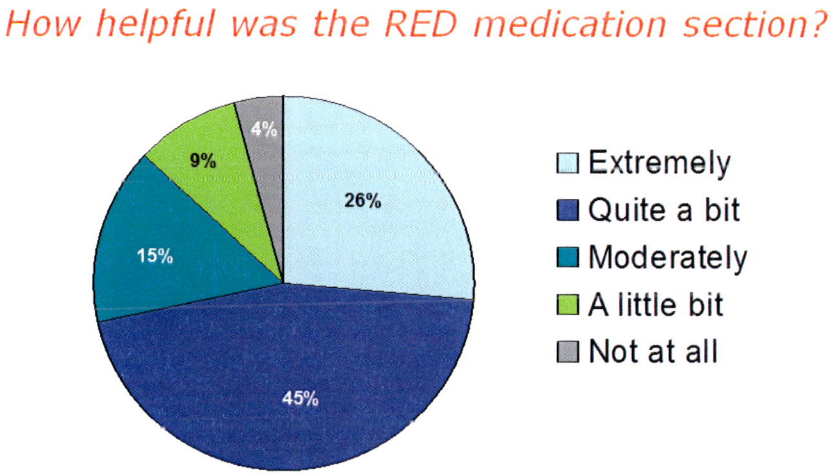

FIGURE 4-6 Evaluation results for the medication section of the after-hospital care plan.
SOURCE: As presented by Brian Jack, November 17, 2016.

hospital care plan showed that a majority of patients found the medication section extremely, quite a bit, or moderately helpful (see Figure 4-6).

Another section of the after-hospital care plan lists the patient's scheduled follow-up appointments with care team members and for laboratory tests (see Figure 4-7). It also includes any delivery scheduled for required medical equipment, such as a hospital bed or oxygen. An accompanying calendar, color coded to correspond to the appointment list, provides another way to make sure the patient and caregivers know about what is in store for the patient over the next 30 days.

Discussing the results of the clinical trial in more detail, Jack explained that the Project RED intervention was effective at reducing rehospitalization rates in patients of all health literacy levels. "Across the board, people found it helpful, and it decreased readmissions," said Jack. He also noted that the intervention performed better than the usual discharge process on secondary outcomes, such as knowing the dates of follow-up appointments and the primary care provider's name, as well as on self-prepared readiness for discharge. He pointed out that the Project RED team conducted these assessments 30 days after discharge, when most patients are not going to remember what happened in the hospital. "They do remember there was something about their discharge that was different and better," he said.

After Hospital Care Plan **John Doe** **10/11/05** RED

*****Bring this Plan to each Appointment*****

MAIN PROBLEM:

Chest Pain

APPOINTMENTS:

Monday, October 31st at 1:30pm	Friday, November 4th at 10:00am	Wednesday, November 9th at 9:30am	Tuesday, November 15th at 11:00am
Dr. Chris Manasseh Primary Care Physician (Doctor)	Dr. Sheilah Bernard Consultant (Cardiologist)	Nutritionist	Cardiac Stress Test
at Harvard St. Community Health Center → Jane will drive	at Boston Medical Center; Doctor's Office Building - 642 → Take cab, use cab voucher	at Boston Medical Center → Take #1 bus	at Boston Medical Center 850 Harrison Ave 4th floor – Cardiac Station → Jane will drive; take parking sticker
For a Follow-up appointment	For a heart appointment	To help with food plan	To check your heart
Office Phone #: 617-825-3400	Office Phone #: 617-638-7490	Office Phone #: 617-555-1234	Office Phone #: 617-555-2345

Tests:

Lab test/Studies done in hospital. Waiting for results.

Lab test/ study name	Date done	Name of clinician to review/location	Day/Date subject will see clinician to discuss results?
Stomach biopsy from endoscopy (stomach test)	October 24, 2005	Dr. Manasseh at Harvard Street CHC	Dr. Manasseh will talk to you about results at your appointment with him on October 31, 2005.

FIGURE 4-7 Appointment schedule in an after-hospital care plan.
SOURCE: As presented by Brian Jack, November 17, 2016.

Since this initial study, Jack and his collaborators have applied Project RED in the various units within their hospital. An inpatient Hospital Consumer Assessment of Healthcare Providers and Systems (HCAHPS) survey administered by Press Ganey showed the intervention produced statistically significant improvements in patient understanding of their discharge instructions compared to patients in the same hospital unit and throughout the hospital over the same time period. "You can raise HCAHPS scores based on the quality of the education related to discharge using the Project RED after-hospital care plan tool," said Jack.

He then noted that the clarity of communication around medicines is more complicated than is often appreciated, particularly when a patient has multiple conditions or multiple complicating factors such as low health literacy and depression. A syndemic, he explained, is the aggregation of two or more diseases in a population in which there is some level of positive biological interaction that exacerbates the negative health effects of any or all of the diseases. To illustrate this, he described Project RED data on the relative risk for all-cause rehospitalization within 30 days of discharge. Commenting on the need to account for syndemics, Jack said, "Ideally, we ought to design the discharge package around medicines and other things to most approximate what the risks are that those patients have to individualize the tools that we give them, and we are working on tools that can do that now."

As an example of how these interactions play out, Jack discussed Project RED data showing the impact of depression on 30-day all-cause readmissions, which increased with the severity of the patient's depression (Cancino et al., 2014). Jack and his colleagues also found that individuals with moderate to severe depression did not understand their diagnosis or their instructions as well as those with mild or no depression. The conclusions from these data, he said, is that it is important to consider factors other than health literacy when designing materials and the type of education patients will receive. He and his colleagues are now conducting a clinical trial on patients with mild or moderate depression based on their Patient Health Questionaire-9 scores.

The Project RED postdischarge mediation process map (see Figure 4-8) provides a means of identifying where to measure failure models and analyze the effects of this process. For example, patients do not receive their prescriptions 2 percent of the time at his hospital. In total, about half of the patients are doing something incorrectly with the medications when questioned within 2 days of discharge. He noted that he has stories for each of the failure modes between the many steps of this process. As

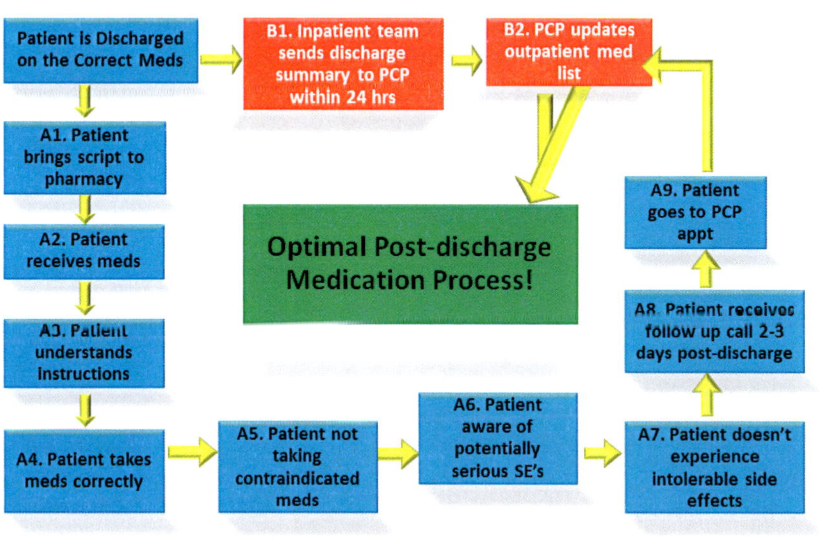

FIGURE 4-8 Project RED postdischarge mediation process map.
NOTE: PCP = primary care provider; SE = side effect.
SOURCE: As presented by Brian Jack, November 17, 2016.

an example, one patient came to his office with materials he had received with his discharge instructions that did not conform to the Project RED requirements. Not only was it nearly illegible, but the instructions were in Latin. "We go to school for years to know what medicine is used for a diagnosis, but we go in a room and spend 2 or 3 or 4 or 5 minutes, and expect somehow magically that people are going to understand all that," said Jack. "This workshop is such an important meeting because the tools that we need to develop are possible, and patients really deserve to know what to do, they want to know what to do, when they go home about how to care for themselves."

Jack concluded his presentation with a brief discussion of Project ACHIEVE Qualitative Analysis, a new project funded by the Patient-Centered Outcomes Research Institute. This 3- to 4-year project is attempting to identify what components of transition in care are important and for whom, he explained. In the study's first year, he and his colleagues conducted 35 focus groups with 96 patients and 75 caregivers as well as 72 key informant interviews with an additional 33 patients and 39 caregivers, producing 2,000 pages of transcripts. What these activities found was that communication, anticipation of needs, and continuity of care are the three main themes for improving care transitions. Communications, for example, have to be purposeful, supportive, and collaborative, according to the patients and caregivers.

Summarizing the results of Project RED, Jack said it improves transitions of care from hospital to home, with the after-hospital care plan serving as the "active ingredient." Project RED benefits those with low health literacy and recognizes that depressive symptoms and other comorbidities impact the ability to understand discharge instructions. Outcomes important to patients and caregivers include communication that is purposeful, supportive, and collaborative, and as a final note, he added that the syndemics of health literacy is an area in which the health literacy field needs to do more work.

PLANNING FOR NON-ENGLISH–SPEAKING PATIENTS[6]

By Charles Lee's estimates, more than 30 million people in the United States do not speak English well, and this group of patients is going to be among the most likely to experience medication errors. He recounted how he used to give medication instruction sheets to some of his patients and they would nod their heads yes when he asked if they understood the

[6] This section is based on the presentation by Charles Lee, president and founder of Polyglot Systems, and the statements are not endorsed or verified by the National Academies of Sciences, Engineering, and Medicine.

instructions. "But they would get that glassy look in their eyes because they really did not understand," said Lee. In his experience, the information he gives patients is the last thing they worry about when under the stress of being discharged and worrying about transportation and other realities of daily life. "What happens is they go home and if they cannot understand the information that is on the handout that's given to them, they have to kind of figure things out, and I think we can do a lot better job," said Lee.

Lee started Polyglot Systems in 2001 and with a Small Business Innovation Research grant from the National Institute on Minority Health and Health Disparities, began to address this issue by developing medication instructions for 120 medications in 6 languages. The focus of this work is to develop a simpler, practical medication monograph, individual instructions for use, a regimen summary based on a visual daily calendar, and 3- to 5-minute video demonstrations on how to use more complex medications. "If you ever try to teach someone to use an inhaler or an eye dropper over the phone with an interpreter, you really cannot," said Lee.

His perspective on health literacy is that it involves three phases: gathering information, understanding it, and acting on it. Given that health literacy is a personal skill and that Polyglot Systems is a small company, his goal is not to teach people how to be more health literate, but rather to leverage information technology to consolidate information, reduce its reading level, and put it in an appropriate language while focusing on key messages, removing clutter, and reducing noise. "We can give them verbal information by video, reinforced in their language, and we can include pictograms for visual referencing, particularly for dosing," said Lee. He noted that his one criticism of FDA's recommendation to limit medication information sheets to one page is that it restricts the ability to use large fonts that may be appropriate for elderly or visually impaired individuals.

Another emphasis of his work is to provide patients with language-appropriate materials that recommend specific actions, such as a calendar with dates and times at which patients need to take their medications. He also stressed the importance of producing materials that encourage dialogue with pharmacists and health care providers and that are individualized for each patient. Regarding this last point, Lee said that many drug monographs include information relevant to multiple indications that patients then need to sift through to find the information specific to their particular medical issue.

The biggest challenge in this work, said Lee, was working with consumer medication information sheets in English. "We are creating materials that people are not reading and it made no sense translating them into documents that nobody is going to read," said Lee. "What we had to do was start with simplifying the English." He showed one example of the company's "Meducation" drug information sheet that illustrates how to

Para ver esta información en Internet o en otros idiomas, vaya a www.meducation.com.

meducation®

0 2 Z J Y R T Q

UNIVERSITY MEDICAL CENTER
University Medical Center
123 Main Street
Anytown, NC 12345
212-555-2121

Biaxin Oral Suspension 125 mg/5 mL

Este medicamento se usa para tratar infecciones.

Cómo tomar el medicamento

Tome el medicamento por la boca dos veces al día con las comidas - desayuno y cena.
Take the medicine by mouth twice a day with meals - breakfast and dinner.

Tome 5 cc (ml) cada vez.
Drink 5 mL each time.

Desayuno	Almuerzo	Comida	Al acostarse
5 cc		5 cc	

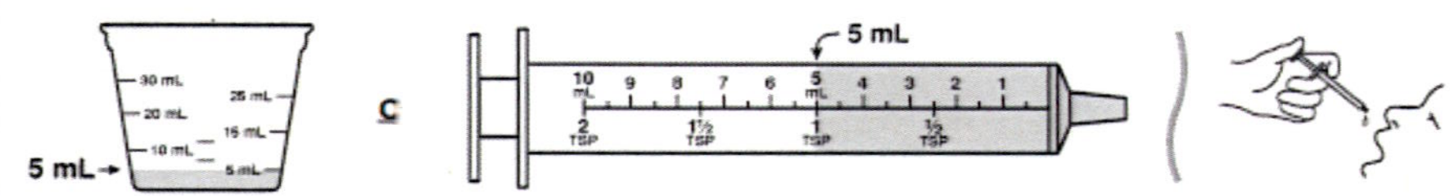

mL = cc

Use el medicamento por 10 días en total.

Instrucciones

Tome el medicamento con alimentos.

Mantenga este medicamento a temperatura ambiente.

Agite la botella bien antes de tomar esta medicamento.

Evite beber jugo de toronja o pomelo mientras esté tomando este medicamento.

Una vez que haya tomado el medicamento por el número total de días indicados, deseche todo el medicamento restante.

Es importante que continúe tomando todas las dosis de este medicamento a la hora indicada aunque se sienta bien.

Si olvida tomar una dosis, tómela tan pronto como se acuerde. Si es casi hora de su siguiente dosis, en lugar de tomar la dosis olvidada vuelva a su programa regular. No tome 2 dosis de este medicamento a la vez.

Informe a su médico o farmacéutico si usted toma algún otro medicamento con o sin receta, vitaminas, medicamentos herbales o alguna otra cosa para su salud.

Ref#: 02ZJYRTQ-92537	Spanish
02/19/2014	Biaxin Oral Suspension 125 mg/5 mL (1 of 2)

FIGURE 4-9 A sample Polyglot Systems Meducation drug information sheet.
SOURCE: As presented by Charles Lee, November 17, 2016.

administer an oral antibiotic (see Figure 4-9). This sheet was derived from the drug monography, which does not include use instructions. He noted that the idea behind this sheet is to provide the same information, at a fifth to eighth grade level, that a good pharmacist might provide to an individual in a 2- to 3-minute conversation. "We are not trying to be a comprehensive drug reference source," said Lee. "We are saying, 'For you to use it safely, to know how to store it and discard it, what information do you need?'"

His company has also developed multilanguage discharge instructions that rely on visual drug regimen summaries for clarity (see Figure 4-10). He likened this sheet to a stacked series of uniform medication schedules that shows visually when a patient needs to take each medication throughout the day. If a medicine has a demonstration, this sheet will also include a Quick Response (QR) barcode that patients can scan using their phones to view the demonstration in the appropriate language.

Today, Polyglot Systems produces these instructional materials in more than 20 languages, including both left-to-right and right-to-left languages. Lee showed a video demonstration, accessible on a smart phone, of how

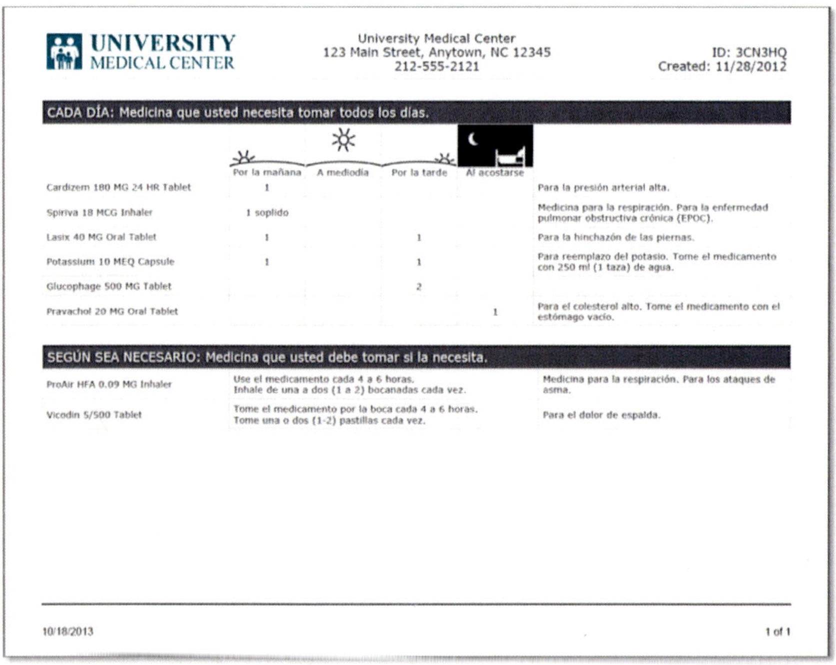
UNIVERSITY MEDICAL CENTER

University Medical Center
123 Main Street, Anytown, NC 12345
212-555-2121

ID: 3CN3HQ
Created: 11/28/2012

CADA DÍA: Medicina que usted necesita tomar todos los días.	Por la mañana	A mediodía	Por la tarde	Al acostarse	
Cardizem 180 MG 24 HR Tablet	1				Para la presión arterial alta.
Spiriva 18 MCG Inhaler	1 soplido				Medicina para la respiración. Para la enfermedad pulmonar obstructiva crónica (EPOC).
Lasix 40 MG Oral Tablet	1		1		Para la hinchazón de las piernas.
Potassium 10 MEQ Capsule	1		1		Para reemplazo del potasio. Tome el medicamento con 250 ml (1 taza) de agua.
Glucophage 500 MG Tablet			2		
Pravachol 20 MG Oral Tablet				1	Para el colesterol alto. Tome el medicamento con el estómago vacío.

SEGÚN SEA NECESARIO: Medicina que usted debe tomar si la necesita.		
ProAir HFA 0.09 MG Inhaler	Use el medicamento cada 4 a 6 horas. Inhale de una a dos (1 a 2) bocanadas cada vez.	Medicina para la respiración. Para los ataques de asma.
Vicodin 5/500 Tablet	Tome el medicamento por la boca cada 4 a 6 horas. Tome una o dos (1-2) pastillas cada vez.	Para el dolor de espalda.

10/18/2013 1 of 1

FIGURE 4-10 Medication discharge instructions to improve medication adherence.
SOURCE: As presented by Charles Lee, November 17, 2016.

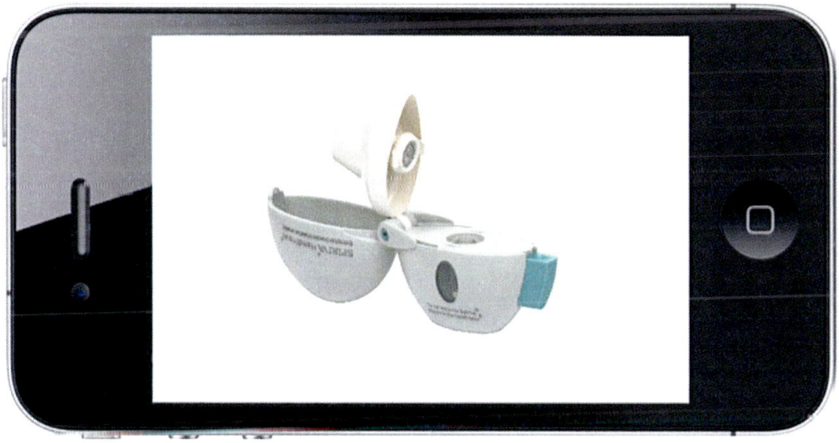

FIGURE 4-11 Mobile patient education for the Spiriva inhaler.
SOURCE: As presented by Charles Lee, November 17, 2016,

to use a Spiriva inhaler, which he said is not an easy device to use (see Figure 4-11). "What has been happening is the patient is in a rush at the pharmacy, they pick up the bag with the box in it, they go home, nobody has taught them how to use this," said Lee. The package contains capsules that the patient is supposed to insert into a plastic inhaler and pierce to inhale the powder, but what some patients are doing is swallowing the capsules, which is the equivalent to not taking the drug at all. "Being able to have instructions they can look at once they go home is important," said Lee.

Creating these materials requires a combination of science and art, said Lee. The science includes all of the findings of health literacy research, including what is known about reading level, visual layouts, font sizes, and the need to reinforce learnings. The art includes deciding on the key points that materials must cover as well as what information to omit. Determining reading level is also an art in that materials at the lowest grade reading level are not always better, Lee explained, because they can lose important nuances. The right reading level, he said, is one that is sufficient to convey the concept and conditions of a particular sentence. Choosing the right visual representations is also more art than science. As an example he said the graphic for food, which would be used to illustrate that a medication needs to be taken with a meal, can range from a piece of pizza to a bowl of rice depending on the cultural background of the intended recipient. "You have to think about universal representations of concepts, which is challenging," he noted.

Label instructions, also known as SIG instructions from the Latin term for "let it be labeled," present a number of challenges. His team has analyzed more than 7 million SIGs from pharmacies and health systems, and most of them are what Lee called free text SIGs, such as "take one tablet by mouth once daily" or "take one table per oral each day," which are two ways of giving the same instruction. The challenge, he explained, comes from the multitude of different permutations of dose, frequency, and indication that make automated translation nearly impossible. Another challenge arises when instructions require the patient to calculate the right dose (e.g., mg to mL), when they are ambiguous, when fractions are involved—is ¼ better than 0.25? For example, the ambiguous instruction "one spray by nasal route daily," could mean one spray in each nostril or one spray in only one nostril. The difference between these two interpretations is a doubling of the dose, explained Lee. In addition, he said, many languages do have concepts for some forms of the drug, such as a softgel or a gelcap.

Pictograms represent a good way of presenting dosing information, particularly as dosing volumes move away from teaspoons and tablespoons to milliliters, but which type of syringe or cup to use in a picture will depend on which device the pharmacy provides to the patient (see Figure 4-12). Tapering instructions as presented today are often too complicated for many patients to follow, and Lee presented a possible alternative that can provide clarity and be easily translated into multiple languages (see Figure 4-13). Similar approaches are needed for non-daily repetitive schedules such as take one pill every other day; different doses on alternating days, such as for warfarin; or varying dosing, as is the case for insulin. All of these, said Lee in closing, are difficult for patients to comprehend and challenging to represent in English, let alone translate into other languages.

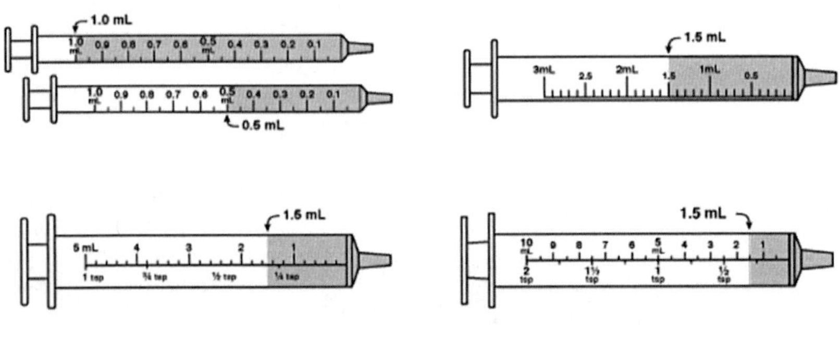

FIGURE 4-12 Different pictograms for illustrating the same dose.
SOURCE: As presented by Charles Lee, November 17, 2016.

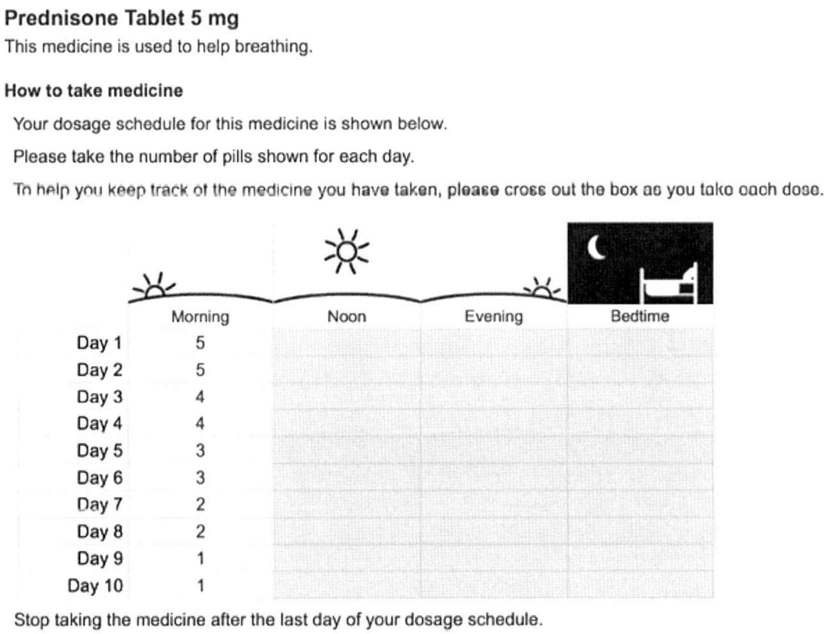

Prednisone Tablet 5 mg

This medicine is used to help breathing.

How to take medicine

Your dosage schedule for this medicine is shown below.

Please take the number of pills shown for each day.

To help you keep track of the medicine you have taken, please cross out the box as you take each dose.

	Morning	Noon	Evening	Bedtime
Day 1	5			
Day 2	5			
Day 3	4			
Day 4	4			
Day 5	3			
Day 6	3			
Day 7	2			
Day 8	2			
Day 9	1			
Day 10	1			

Stop taking the medicine after the last day of your dosage schedule.

FIGURE 4-13 A visual presentation of tapering instructions.
SOURCE: As presented by Charles Lee, November 17, 2016.

REACTOR PANEL COMMENTS[7]

Commenting on the four presentations from the perspective of a retail pharmacist and a member of both the Massachusetts Board of Pharmacy and the National Association of Boards of Pharmacy, Donna Horn noted that Sparks was correct about the challenge of working with pharmacy software vendors, each of which has its own process for generating prescription labels. One thing she sees often with labels is that the directions are in all capital letters, which literacy research has shown makes reading and comprehension difficult. Nonetheless, many vendors sell software that only uses capital letters and getting them to change that would require them

[7] This section is based on the comments of Donna Horn, director of patient safety-community pharmacy at the Institute for Safe Medication Practices, and H. Shonna Yin, associate professor of pediatrics and population health in the Departments of Pediatrics and Population Health at the New York University School of Medicine and Bellevue Hospital Center, and the statements are not endorsed or verified by the National Academies of Sciences, Engineering, and Medicine.

to redesign their programs. "They cannot do that. They [would] have to start from scratch," said Horn.

Label real estate presents another challenge given that state pharmacy boards require a certain amount of information on every label. She suggested that the manufacturer's name and prescribing physician's name could be left off a label without depriving the patient of important information. "We have to look at the information required to be on a label and ask the board of pharmacy what can be taken off to make the label easier to read," Horn suggested.

She also commented on the NVS instrument to test an individual's health literacy, noting that it is impossible to use at the pharmacy. "If you are at CVS or Walgreens or Walmart or Rite Aid or anywhere, no one is going to stop and ask you to do the Newest Vital Sign, even though it's a great test," said Horn. She added that showing the NVS to pharmacists was "really an eye opener for them." Instead of relying on the NVS, she recommended making the information as simple as possible given that nobody will be insulted if medication information is presented to them in simple terms.

One pushback she gets from the pharmacy students she teaches at the Massachusetts College of Pharmacy is that they cannot change what the doctor wrote. For example, while the prescribing physician will write, "take one tablet twice daily," the better instruction would be to tell the patient to take one tablet in the morning and one at night, or take one at breakfast and one at dinner to tie it to something they are going to do as part of their daily routine. The solution, she said, is to work with prescribers to teach them to write health-literate prescriptions in the way they would want the pharmacist to type that information on the label given to patients. When she has done that, it has changed prescribers' minds about how they wrote their prescriptions.

Commenting on the fact that every state requires pharmacists to offer counseling for every new prescription, she noted Lee's remark that the time when most patients have questions is when they start taking a medication, not when the pharmacist is handing it to them with the medication guide that they more than likely throw out when they get home. In addition, many companies have decided to provide that information the first time they fill a prescription, not with subsequent refills. "When the patient actually has a question, the information is not there." The lesson she learned from the presentations, she said, is that it is important to understand that people have questions as they go through the journey of taking their medications.

Horn said she and her colleagues at the Institute for Safe Medication Practices developed a medication leaflet containing the 10 factors that would allow patients to take their medications safely.[8] There is a question, however, about the feasibility of implementing this list, she noted. She also wondered if the Polyglot Systems approach could create individualized labels at the pharmacy and fit into the workflow of the retail pharmacy. She remarked that the idea of putting a QR barcode on a label was interesting, but she worried about their utility for people who are not technologically knowledgeable.

Lee's comment about getting rid of teaspoons and tablespoons is something her organization feels strongly about and is working toward eliminating and replacing with milliliters. Similarly, instructions such as "take one tablet at 10 AM on days one to four of the week," must be replaced, she said, with "take one tablet at 10 AM on Monday and Thursday," for example. "The more we can get that information on the prescription, then we can actually type it onto the label and things will be better for patients," said Horn.

Shonna Yin, a pediatrician who works on designing and evaluating health literacy–informed intervention tools to improve communication between health care providers and families, including communication about medication instructions, began her comments by noting that she is working on a project funded by the National Institutes of Health to redesign medication labels for pediatric liquid medicines. She remarked that each of the presentations in this session provided solutions to important pieces of the medication safety problem, but she worries that few institutions and organizations are implementing these effective programs. "How do we get from where we are now to where we want to be, where all patients are able to receive information that is understandable?" asked Yin. "Is it necessary for us to go state by state battling to get regulations instituted?" She applauded the rigorous approach Sparks has taken in Wisconsin, assessing barriers, creating an advisory council, and getting patient feedback and input, but she questioned whether this same process should have to take place in every state. "It seems like a daunting process that will take us decades before everyone has low-literacy labels," said Yin. "How can we better engage large chain pharmacies that span across states to try to get them to adopt and lead by example? How can we get corporate buy-in and present a business case for health literacy–informed labeling?" She wondered if there was a role for the National Association of Boards of Pharmacy to play in trying to push this issue forward and was optimistic that the upcoming labeling summit in Wisconsin could provide the impetus to push the field forward.

[8] Available at http://www.consumermedsafety.org/tools-and-resources/medication-safety-tools-and-resources/consumer-medsafety-lists/item/537-top-ten-things-you-must-know-about-the-medicine-you-are-taking (accessed March 31, 2017).

Yin noted how impressed she was with Myers's presentation on the work Merck is doing and the company's commitment to health literacy issues, particularly related to how it is involving patients with low health literacy in its development efforts. She wondered if FDA might be able to recommend that all pharmaceutical companies adopt such best practices or push for more standards in terms of testing drug information. "Could the FDA perhaps recommend some minimum number of low-literacy patients, for example, that medication information should be tested with?" she asked. Perhaps the agency could set a goal, she suggested, of having at least 25 percent of the individuals who are involved in testing the comprehensibility of informational materials on drugs be of low health literacy, given that more than half of the U.S. population struggles with health literacy issues. She also wondered if criteria could be established for thresholds of understanding. Referring to Merck's ability to exceed 85 percent comprehension across different health literacy levels, Yin said, "I would love to understand more about how comprehension is tested, and how that could be adopted in other places."

Yin also expressed her admiration for Project RED and the rigor with which Jack and his colleagues approached this problem, and demonstrated the business case of reducing readmissions. She acknowledged that many institutions are now adopting Project RED, but she wishes adoption was happening more widely. She wondered about whether Project RED could be integrated with EHR systems and expanded beyond the discharge process to include regular outpatient encounters or encounters in emergency department settings, as these are also settings where people are being sent home with prescribed medications. She had similar comments about the promise of Meducation and the slow pace of widespread adoption. "I wonder how we can encourage health systems to adopt these interventions more universally and what processes need to be in place to engage those large EHR vendors as a start to get them to adopt these kinds of interventions more broadly," said Yin.

Commenting further on the glacial pace of adoption, she noted that despite concrete recommendations on health literacy–informed layout and content, as well as evidence-based interventions and FDA efforts to try to incorporate health literacy principles across the agency, widespread adoption of these approaches is not happening. Leveraging technology to increase adoption will be important, she said. She also pointed out that digital interoperability still has a long way to go to better coordinate the information being given out by physicians and pharmacists. "There is no cohesiveness in the messages," she said, hoping that a consolidated portal could be used as a single source from which patients, family members, and other caregivers would receive information seamlessly.

Noting her disappointment at how often medication information is not available in a patient's primary language and the poor quality of translations that many patients are able to access, Yin asked if there could be an information bank that would house well-thought-out translations that any organization could use. "Why is it that every organization, every health system, every EHR vendor, every producer of patient information has to address these issues in their individual silos?" she asked. Despite the challenges, she said she is hopeful that the many stakeholders affected by this issue will be able to develop a plan to move the field forward more quickly.

DISCUSSION

Bernard Rosof opened the discussion by suggesting that wrapping a learning health system around the interventions discussed by the panelists might achieve the more rapid dissemination that Yin discussed. He also noted that because medication health literacy is a systems property, perhaps dissemination might benefit from an examination of the systems in place that might better enable dissemination. As an example, he recounted how he went to his internist, who has been his primary care physician for 15 years, during an episode of dizziness. One thing led to another, and he ended up in the hospital being seen by one specialist after another. After being discharged, he wondered if any of what he had experienced had been communicated with his internist. His question for the panelists was how it would be possible to create an integrated system that would enable the interventions discussed during this session, when even the most integrated delivery systems do not have such systems in place.

Jack replied that the situation Rosof described happens every day, and patients told similar stories when he and his colleagues were conducting focus groups at the start of Project RED. He heard stories about patients being prescribed two different medications by two clinicians for two different conditions, taking their medications properly, and then experiencing a life-threatening complication such as kidney failure resulting from drug–drug interactions. These stories, said Jack, point to the importance of better managing the ever-more-complicated transitions to, within, and from the hospital. Indeed, the goal of Project RED was to do just that for the hospital-to-home transition as a way of addressing the fact that 20 percent of patients who left Boston hospitals were having an adverse event within 20 days of discharge and that nearly 20 percent of Medicare patients are readmitted to the hospital within 30 days. He noted that the postdischarge phone call, which Project RED introduced, is not a social call, but involves the pharmacist asking the patient or caregiver to bring their medications to the phone and reviewing how and when to take them. This step, he said, is critical for identifying potential medication issues of the sort that will lead to expensive rehospitalization.

Horn raised the issue of how problems with information transfer can lead to medication errors. For example, when a patient receives a prescription at the time of discharge, they may go to the hospital pharmacy, where the pharmacist has the ability to review the patient's EHR for any potential problems. However, if the patient decides to have that prescription filled at her local pharmacy, the pharmacist there has no way to look for any additional information. In fact, prescriptions arriving at the pharmacy electronically often need to be transcribed, creating the potential for error. "So once you get the hospital part fixed, you have to bring it back to the local pharmacy, too," said Horn.

Sparks added that transitions from the emergency department and urgent care settings to home are also problematic. In a recent project in which he participated, he was surprised to learn that the urgent care centers belonging to a large health system in Wisconsin did not even provide discharge instructions beyond a few quick verbal instructions even when given prescriptions. "No wonder people forget what they have to do, and some of these folks end up back in the hospital," said Sparks. He recounted one case in which a woman went to the emergency department on a Friday complaining of severe constipation and some digestive problems. She received verbal instructions to go to the drug store to get Prilosec, which she and her husband assumed was a prescription medication. When her husband went to the pharmacy, there was no prescription waiting for him to pick up, so he went home without any medication and his wife was back in the emergency department on Monday.

Cindy Brach from AHRQ asked the panelists for their thoughts on why adoption of more health-literate labels is lagging. Sparks said he believes the reason is that there is no advocacy for this to happen. He told how the pharmacists he has interviewed are all supportive of the USP standards for clearer labels and typically respond with a comment such as, "Well, why would you not want to make a medication label easier to understand?" Nonetheless, this is a back-burner issue for most pharmacists and it will remain so, he predicted, until some organization such as the National Association of State Boards of Pharmacy takes on an advocacy role on this issue.

Jack commented that when he first presented Project RED to the senior management group of his hospital, the chief financial officer wanted to know why decreasing emergency department visits and rehospitalizations was something good given the negative impact that would have on the hospital's operating profits. "As long as we are in a fee-for-service system, even though there are these penalties, the penalties are not nearly big enough to make up for the difference in decrease in hospitalization rates significantly, so there is not much effort happening in many places," said Jack. He also noted that many hospital administrators want to know how to decrease readmissions so that when the financial incentives to do so change, they will be ready to implement programs such as Project RED. Jack was critical, too, of the EHR vendors who in his opinion have done little to improve the discharge instructions their systems produce even though programs are available that could be integrated into EHR systems to produce patient-centered, health-literate documents. As a result, what happens today is that nurses typically have to duplicate discharge information in the Project RED forms, an inefficient process.

Michael Wolf commented that he has been hearing this same conversation for a decade and believes that policies and a reluctance to move forward are the major barriers to adoption of the many proven approaches to producing health-literate medication information. "How much evidence base do you actually have to have before you can allow the ability to be able to go forth and launch something?" he asked. His hope is that health systems will "get out of the way," and allow innovation to occur. "Let us not be so risk averse when we know that much of what we currently do right now, many of our practices, are harmful, and that evidence has shown that people are misinterpreting, making mistakes, and having impacts on their behaviors," said Wolf. He then asked Lee and Jack if they have continual evaluations of their programs to enable continuous improvement. Lee said his company does do that kind of evaluation and improvement, and agreed with Jack's comments that bottom-line issues are a barrier to widespread implementation of these systems. "To me, this is just common sense and it is the right thing to do, but it is surprising how the right thing to do does not get people to move," said Lee. "It has got to hit their bottom line, affect their HCAHPS [Hospital Consumer Assessment of Healthcare Providers and Systems] scores, affect their penalties, and increase revenue, because if they just see this as work and expense, then they will not do it." He added that getting pharmacists and physicians to buy in will require top-down and regulatory pressure.

Lee then explained how Dignity Health, the largest nonprofit hospital system in California, is integrating Polyglot Systems' program into its Cerner EHR. This EHR tracks a patient's preferred language upon admission, and at discharge it sends a reconciled medication list and the preferred language to Polyglot Systems, which then automatically generates the medication list in the appropriate language to be handed to the patient and used to explain the patient's medication regimen. He noted that when San Francisco General Hospital did a pilot study with his company's tool, the readmission rate fell from 26 percent to 8 percent.

Myers said one impediment to scaling these systems is that there are only two people in industry that she knows of—herself and Lori Hall at Eli Lilly and Company—who work full time on health literacy and medication issues. Legal issues are also a barrier in many organizations, she added.

An unidentified participant commented that a study she participated in measured 177 internal medicine patients' understanding in three domains: their diagnosis, medication, and the procedures they experienced when being admitted. There was less than 55 percent concordance between the physicians' documentation and the patients' understanding, even though 45 percent of the patients had at least a college degree. To her, those data point to the implications of health literacy beyond medication issues. She then asked Jack how clinical staff find the time to do the comprehensive work it takes to increase patient understanding. Jack replied that today, the total amount of time that all clinical staff combined spends talking to patients when they go home is in the range of 6 to 8 minutes. Given that most hospitalized patients are not at peak cognitive performance when discharged, Jack said it was "magical thinking" to believe that 6 to 8 minutes is enough time for patients to understand their medications. "That is why written materials are so important and patient caregivers are so important, and why materials that both patient and the caregiver can actually understand are essential," said Jack. His solution is to re-engineer the hospital ward, stop using procedures that are not evidence based, and start using procedures that are evidence based. He noted that he and his colleagues have created an information technology system called Louise that teaches the after-hospital care plans. In a study of 158 patients who used Louise, the patients preferred receiving information from Louise by a two-to-one margin over a doctor or a nurse. The reason the patients gave for that preference was always the same, said Jack: the doctors and nurses were too busy to spend the necessary time.

Wilma Alvarado-Little asked the panelists if they were considering the deaf and hard of hearing and the limited English-proficiency communities in their work. The honest answer, said Myers, is that the field is evolving and continuing to refine its research efforts to include these other communities. She acknowledged that Merck's studies have not yet included anyone from the deaf community. She did note that a number of people for whom English is not their first language have participated in Merck's health literacy studies. Sparks said that USP standards do mention dealing with people who are visually impaired or hard of hearing, but that the expense of installing a system appropriate for those individuals is too high for most pharmacies.

Jack recounted a conversation he had with someone whose hospitalized family member was blind. The patient's room had a large sign above the bed that read, "The patient is blind," and the nurses and other staff were terrific about explaining things verbally. However, at discharge the patient was handed a bunch of paper instructions. He noted that the Louise system is verbal and provides the patient with a CD that they can take home and listen to as needed. He added that there are companies that are developing verbal discharge instruction tools and that the 12th element of Project RED is language assistance, which includes a tool to assess and deliver discharge information for people with various limitations.

Lee remarked that interpreters and translators have told him that they want to stay on the wards and talk to patients, not go to the pharmacy to hand-translate documents. This preference has informed his company's approach to having discharge materials preprinted so the interpreter could review that information with the patient. "This was designed to complement oral interpretation and not replace it," said Lee.

Jennifer Dillaha with the Arkansas Department of Health remarked that her state has a large rural population and that when patients are discharged, they can be quite far from the hospital once they return home. To address this problem, Arkansas has been looking at establishing better linkages between hospitals and local primary care physicians as well as community paramedic programs and home health care agencies. She asked the panelists if they had any experience with such efforts and how they might affect medication adherence. Lee replied that one issue is dealing with the portability of the medication lists across transitions of care. The Office of the National Coordinator for Health Information Technology, he explained, is working with EHR vendors on a universal or centralized up-to-date medication list. One challenge this effort is facing is the need to incorporate a feature that would allow patients and the home care nurse to provide input to the medication list. The degree to which solutions can be focused around the patient is critical to address the problem Dillaha described, said Lee.

Sparks noted that involving community paramedics is an excellent idea. He explained that he has had the opportunity to provide health literacy training to community paramedics and believes these professionals need to understand and be skilled in health literacy techniques, something that is currently the exception rather than the rule.

5

Exploring the Future of Health-Literate Design

The workshop's final panel session featured three presentations on the future of health-literate design. Daniel Morrow, chair of the Department of Educational Psychology at the University of Illinois at Urbana-Champaign, discussed the changing ecology of medication information for patients and how Web-based information can be improved to help increase patient understanding. Heather Rennie, managing counsel in the Regulatory Legal Group at Merck Sharp & Dohme Corp., then provided a lawyer's perspective on health literacy and medication information. Next, Michael Wolf, professor of medicine and learning disease and associate division chief for research in the Division of General Internal Medicine at Northwestern University's Feinberg School of Medicine, provided his view of the future of health literacy research as applied to written medication communications. An open discussion moderated by Bernard Rosof followed the three presentations.

WRITTEN MATERIALS IN THE DIGITAL SPACE[1]

Daniel Morrow began the first presentation of the session by reminding the participants that there is a changing ecology of health information that may have implications for the cognitive accessibility of this information,

---

[1] This section is based on the presentation by Daniel Morrow, chair of the Department of Educational Psychology at the University of Illinois at Urbana-Champaign, and the statements are not endorsed or verified by the National Academies of Sciences, Engineering, and Medicine.

particularly for older adults (Sharit et al., 2008). Traditionally, health information has been paper based, and for chronically ill or elderly patients, who may be taking multiple medications, the paper burden can be substantial. Today, that situation is evolving into one in which patients are getting their medication information via patient portals and other Web-based sources and are managing their medications with the help of electronic tools such as mobile phones or tablet apps. This new electronic ecology, as opposed to a written ecology, affords opportunities to increase patient access and comprehension while also constraining how individuals understand health information (Czaja et al., 2013; Taha et al., 2013, 2014).

With regard to access, Morrow explained there are challenges related to the digital divide, but also with cognitive abilities as much as technology access. The act of reading, for example, is changing, where patients are browsing electronic material more than they used to when receiving information on paper. Reading, he said, is less of a linear act when done online. People are also managing multiple documents online, perhaps guided by hyperlinks and search engines, and they have the opportunity to benefit from multimedia approaches to information dissemination. All of these factors, he said, change the requirements for comprehension substantially and place more emphasis on integrating information across multiple documents and search results.

Learning is always to some extent self-regulated, said Morrow, but it is even more so in an electronic environment. When getting information online, without having anyone present to assist them, individuals have to self-monitor whether they are truly understanding what they are reading, whether they can evaluate information to make intelligent decisions about where to go next, and how to integrate information from the multiple sources they may find in their web searches. This challenge, he said, is likely to be even greater for older adults, who may not only be less comfortable with or knowledgeable about getting information electronically, but also less cognitively able to process that information because of age-related changes in literacy and cognitive abilities (Czaja et al., 2013; Sharit et al., 2008; Taha et al., 2014).

Morrow then discussed the work he and his colleagues have been using to try to help older adults better understand both paper and electronic information. The first step, he said, is to identify the cognitive resources and abilities people need to understand health information. Next comes an analysis of how those resources and abilities influence comprehension processes and whether those processes differ in an electronic versus paper environment. These analyses can provide a firmer scientific basis for developing interventions targeted to fixing the identified problems.

This approach relies heavily on the large body of research on how aging affects cognition and how health literacy ties into that process. "For understanding the processes of comprehension, we rely on theories of text processing, language comprehension, multimedia comprehension processes, and then these same theories may help us come up with innovative solutions, design-based solutions," Morrow said. He explained that like many researchers in the field, including Wolf and Ruth Parker, he looks at health literacy as a function involving the resources that patients bring to health care and the demands on those resources that self-care tasks such as taking medication require (see Figure 5-1). This approach leads to a focus on processing capacity and working memory processing speed in relation to aging.

To make this theoretical approach more tangible, Morrow reviewed some of the cognitive work that occurs to understand the seemingly simple instruction to take one tablet every day. First, the individual has to recognize the words. That recognition activates nodes in a mental dictionary encompassing that person's understanding of associated concepts. That alone, however, is not sufficient for comprehension, so the next step is to put concepts together to understand the idea the sentence is conveying. In this case, that sentence is conveying an action involving a number of tablets at a specific frequency. "You put those concepts together to get a sense of the basic concept of the sentence, and that will take you some way toward comprehension, but certainly not all the way," said Morrow. What has to

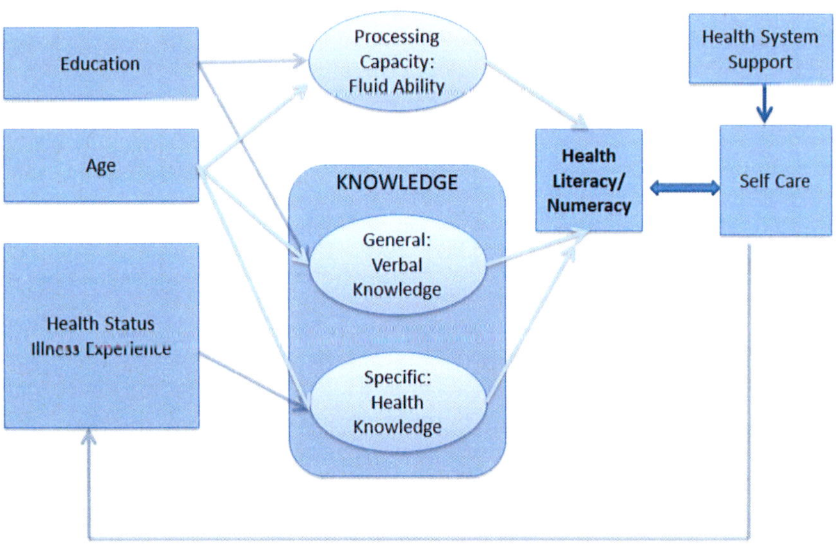

FIGURE 5-1 The process/knowledge model of health literacy.
SOURCES: As presented by Daniel Morrow, November 17, 2016. From Chin et al., 2011.

happen, he explained, is for the mind to elaborate on the mental representation of those ideas with knowledge about medication and from other domains to arrive at a mental or situational model of the task at hand. This is in essence a mental simulation, Morrow said.

In the context of this model, aging is associated with reduced processing capacity, a constraint that makes those component processes harder, less efficient, and less accurate. At the same time, knowledge accumulated over a lifetime of encounters with health care systems can make those processes easier, more efficient, and more accurate. That last assumption may be less true, he added, for individuals with low health literacy compared to those with high health literacy. Morrow is now trying to decompose health literacy into age-related concepts that may interact in terms of how they influence comprehension, decision making, and self-care behavior. "The action is in the interplay of processing capacity constraints and knowledge-based facilitation," he explained.

As an example of research results that are consistent with this model, he and his colleagues found that older adults' ability to recall hypertension information was predicted by the Short Test of Functional Health Literacy in Adults (Chin et al., 2015), an unsurprising result, he said, given that other investigators have made similar observations. Further analysis allowed them to account for much of the relationship between this health literacy measure and recall in terms of processing capacity and knowledge. The interactions among these components were also important for predicting outcomes, he added. This analysis also suggests that the ability to learn self-care information can be improved by reducing the demands of learning on processing capacity and by leveraging knowledge to support learning.

Regarding the second stage in the three-stage model—analyzing how resources influence self-care processes—Morrow explained that a large body of evidence has shown that people have a harder time recognizing longer, less familiar words, which in practical terms means that jargon represents a design challenge when creating health-literate information. Concept integration is also influenced negatively by lower health literacy resources, leading to poorer memory of information. Low health literacy also impairs an individual's ability to elaborate concepts with knowledge, which means that poorly organized text or complex or irrelevant graphics may undermine comprehension, particularly in digital environments, said Morrow.

He concluded his presentation by discussing an intervention study in which he and his colleagues were trying to target particular comprehension processes and reduce demands on cognitive resources, thereby helping people leverage knowledge they have to improve comprehension. This intervention was a multifaceted approach to redesigning Web based information for self-care of hypertension. This effort started with finding good examples of information about hypertension from reliable sources such as the Mayo

Clinic and the National Institutes of Health, among others. Guided by their theories and earlier findings, Morrow and his collaborators developed a comprehensive multilevel approach to improve comprehension and memory of the information from these sources. Working with medical specialists, behavioral scientists, computer scientists, and patients, they went through all of the information systematically to identify which information was needed for maximum understanding while also thinking about how to use familiar concepts to help leverage preexisting knowledge. They also focused on simplifying language and sentence structure in ways that might help older adults who have a great deal of literacy experience and on how to organize information logically rather than in the disjointed manner that was common in the materials they found in their initial search. Research Morrow had conducted in the past had shown that patients want information in a particular order and flow, so his team was careful about the titles, headers, and advance organizers it used in the materials it was creating.

Once the redesign of information was complete, Morrow's team had 128 people read both the original and revised passages on a computer at their own pace and then summarize the main points and answer a set of questions about explicitly presented and inferred concepts. The readers had a mean age of 71 years and a high school education or less.

Test subjects remembered the revised passages more accurately, said Morrow, and required less effort to understand the same amount of information and understand both inferred and explicit concepts. Older adults with more health knowledge benefited more from the revised passages. Morrow said the most important piece of the redesign, particularly for older adults, was reorganizing content and systematically signaling how the information was going to be conveyed. Reorganizing content may also support self-regulated learning experiences, he said in closing, by making the process of remembering key concepts more efficient, thus freeing cognitive resources to evaluate comprehension in the context of online environments.

LEGAL CONSIDERATIONS IN APPLYING HEALTH LITERACY PRINCIPLES TO WRITTEN COMMUNICATION[2]

The health literacy world has the perception that lawyers are an obstacle to health literacy, said Heather Rennie as an introduction to her presentation. "I am here to tell you that is not the case, certainly not at Merck," she said. "But it is important for you to understand how lawyers think and how that might be perceived as a block when you talk to lawyers

[2] This section is based on the presentation by Heather Rennie, managing counsel of the Regulatory Legal Group at Merck Sharp & Dohme Corp., and the statements are not endorsed or verified by the National Academies of Sciences, Engineering, and Medicine.

about health literacy." Certainly, she acknowledged, legalese—an English term first used in 1914 to describe legal writing designed to be difficult for common people to read and understand—does conflict with the notion of health literacy.

From a lawyer's perspective, words matter, and a lawyer's job is to ensure that what is said will be found to mean precisely what is intended upon later scrutiny, Rennie explained. A lawyer, she added, must be aware not only of the natural meaning of the words, but also of the special meaning such words may have acquired by legal convention and by previous decisions of the courts. "What does this mean in terms of health literacy?" she asked. "Someone said earlier today to keep it simple, but whenever you get lawyers involved, they are going to want to add words because they are going to want to make sure that they have covered everything, and so sometimes that makes things difficult when you think about health literacy and prescription drug labeling."

In contrast to what one might believe, the primary purpose of prescription drug labeling is not to give patients the information they need to take medications properly, said Rennie. Although patients may obtain useful information from prescription drug labeling, its primary purpose is to give health care professionals the information they need to prescribe the drugs appropriately, which Rennie said is an important distinction to remember. "Fundamentally, prescription drug labeling is designed first and foremost for the health care professionals who are making the prescribing decisions," she said. Given that, she listed a number of general requirements for prescription drug labeling:

- summary of the safe and effective use of the drug
- informative and accurate
- not promotional, false, or misleading
- no implied claims or suggestions for use if evidence of safety or effectiveness is lacking
- based whenever possible on data derived from human experience
- approved by the U.S. Food and Drug Administration (FDA)

Current forms of patient labeling that are part of FDA-approved prescription drug labeling include package patient inserts, which are approved by FDA and are required only for certain classes of medicines; instructions for use, also approved by FDA and required for medicines with complicated dosing instructions; and medication guides, again approved by FDA and required under certain circumstances such as when a product has serious adverse events associated with its use or when adherence to directions is crucial to the product's effectiveness. The regulations governing prescription drug labeling encompass health literacy principles, said Rennie. Medication guides, for example, must be written in nontechnical, understandable language that is scientifically accurate, based on and not in conflict with the professional labeling for the product, and not promotional in nature.

FDA regulations also govern drug promotional materials, Rennie explained, and the information in these materials must be consistent with the approved product labeling. Promotional materials intended for physicians, for example, have to be consistent with the physician prescribing information, while consumer-directed materials must be consistent with approved patient labeling. Promotional materials must be supported by substantial evidence, balance efficacy, and risk information; must include all material information; and must not be false or misleading. As a regulatory lawyer, Rennie looks at materials that come through Merck's Promotional Review Committee for consistency between physician prescribing information and patient product information. "In fact, I am going to look for the language to be identical," she said.

From a health literacy standpoint, this means that if health literacy concepts are not incorporated from the start, it will be difficult for her as the regulatory attorney to become comfortable approving materials that change language appearing in the FDA-approved label. She also has to think about product liability because if a patient has an adverse event, they may want to sue the company or the prescriber. An important concept in product liability, Rennie explained, is the learned intermediary rule. In most jurisdictions, there is a defense for failure-to-warn claims that relieves a pharmaceutical company of its duty to warn the patient if the manufacturer supplying the drug provides information to the physician about the drug's dangerous properties. What this means is that the physician acts as a learned intermediary between the manufacturer and consumer and is liable for any damages resulting from use of a drug for which the physician received notice of possible adverse events.

The rationale for this doctrine, said Rennie, is that the entire U.S. system of drug distribution is set up to place the responsibility of distribution and use on professional people. Reflecting that idea, laws and regulations prevent prescription drugs from being purchased by individuals without the advice, guidance, and consent of licensed physicians and pharmacists. "These professionals are in the best position to evaluate the warnings put out by the drug industry," said Rennie. "As a medical expert, the prescribing physician can take into account the propensities of the drug as well as the susceptibilities of the patient, and I would argue the health literacy of the patient."

New Jersey, Rennie noted, has an exception to this rule known as the direct-to-consumer advertising exception. In New Jersey, pharmaceutical companies that market directly to consumers can be held liable on a failure-to-warn claim. "However, even in New Jersey, if your promotional materials disclose the risks that are included in your patient labeling—if they comply with the language in your patient product labeling—the manufacturer is discharged from liability," said Rennie.

She noted that one could argue that the current state of product liability law is a disincentive to health literacy from a pharmaceutical company perspective, but she does not believe that to be true. "I think it is still incumbent upon pharmaceutical companies to make sure patients understand the risks and benefits of the product, but certainly the learned intermediary doctrine places the onus on the prescribing physician because it is viewed that the prescribing physician is in the best place to have the discussion with the patient and to know their particular circumstances," said Rennie.

From a legal perspective, health literacy must be considered in product labeling, and while legal considerations may present challenges, they are not insurmountable. Timing is important and should be considered from the start of product labeling, though labels are updated if a safety issue arises in the course of postmarketing surveillance. "You can take health literacy into context then, too," said Rennie. For products that have been on the market for a long time without any label changes, it is important to determine where the best opportunities exist to incorporate health literacy. Certainly, she said, there are no issues with reformatting labeling materials to reflect health literacy principles, nor are there legal issues with updating disease-related information to reflect new knowledge.

Rennie concluded her presentation by calling for everyone—health care professionals, the pharmaceutical industry, regulators, lawyers, and patients—to work together. "If you have lawyers in your organization and they are not at the table with you, you should bring them to the table because when the lawyers understand what you are trying to accomplish, they will help you find a solution."

MOVING FORWARD IN WRITTEN COMMUNICATIONS RESEARCH[3]

Michael Wolf began the session's final presentation by thanking Cindy Brach in her role at the Agency for Healthcare Research and Quality (AHRQ) for being a great advocate for much of the work discussed at this workshop. He then reminded the participants that the Institute of Medicine started thinking about standardizing medication labels in 2007

[3] This section is based on the presentation by Michael Wolf, professor of medicine and learning disease and associate division chief for research in the Division of General Internal Medicine at Northwestern University's Feinberg School of Medicine, and the statements are not endorsed or verified by the National Academies of Sciences, Engineering, and Medicine.

(IOM, 2008), and in the decade since that first effort, there have been some hard-fought wins. The health literacy field, he noted, has built a sizable. research-generated evidence base related to medication materials (Bailey et al., 2015; Shrank et al., 2007). FDA and U.S. Pharmacopeia (USP) have become valuable contributors to this work, as have The Brookings Institution and the Margolis Center for Health Policy at Duke University.

Wolf said he was excited to hear during the workshop about the continued expansion of policy reform in several states being spearheaded by state boards of pharmacy, which are working together to push through meaningful changes intended to get a better label with better information to patients. He acknowledged the support for these efforts from the National Association of Boards of Pharmacy, too, as well as high-level engagement by the pharmaceutical industry involving people who are trying to find a way to do better at helping people use their medications. "I think it is important for us to recognize that we have done a great deal of good in a short period of time," said Wolf.

Nonetheless, there are a number of issues at the intersection of health literacy and medication misuse that research has identified and that the field needs to address, said Wolf. These include

- reconciling medications;
- spacing out multidaily dosing;
- remembering to take medication, a particular problem for low health literacy patients;
- organizing and integrating complex prescription regimens; and
- problem solving, such as learning about side effects and knowing what actions to take if a dose is missed or a medication is misused.

Wolf then discussed the findings from a recent systematic review of interventions to improve medication information for low health literacy populations (Wali et al., 2016). This review of some 50 published papers examined interventions in six categories—written information, visual information, audible or verbal information, label information, reminder systems, and education programs and services. While the majority of the evidence in the reviewed studies was "mediocre," according to Wolf, about half to two-thirds of the studies in each of the six categories were successful at improving comprehension, with a few interventions improving medication adherence or behavioral outcomes. The most important finding from this review, however, was that the best interventions were not singular in their approach, but were supported by tailored, personalized materials from other sources. For example, a patient receiving verbal counseling would also receive written materials specific to the individual that supported the spoken message. In addition, interventions that targeted health systems to ease navigation and simplify access to content also were the most successful, explained Wolf.

A decade ago, Wolf continued, he and colleagues Terry Davis, Ruth Parker, and Alastair Wood proposed what would eventually be called the Universal Medication Schedule (UMS). The basic idea of the UMS (see Figure 5-2), he explained, was to write instructions more explicitly using a construct that individuals at any level of health literacy would understand. A recently published study (Wolf et al., 2016), funded by AHRQ, showed that the UMS had a modest effect on improving adherence among the general population, but had a more substantial effect on individuals with limited literacy skills who were taking more complex drug regimens or who had medications prescribed for multidaily dosing. Given the low cost of implementing the UMS on written instructions, he predicted the benefit-to-cost ratio for the UMS would be large.

The evidence generated so far on the effectiveness of various interventions on medication adherence and safe use has produced a few important takeaways, said Wolf. The first is that plain language in written prescription drug labeling alone has a limited ability to reduce disparities among individuals with low literacy. "That is just a statement," said Wolf. "It

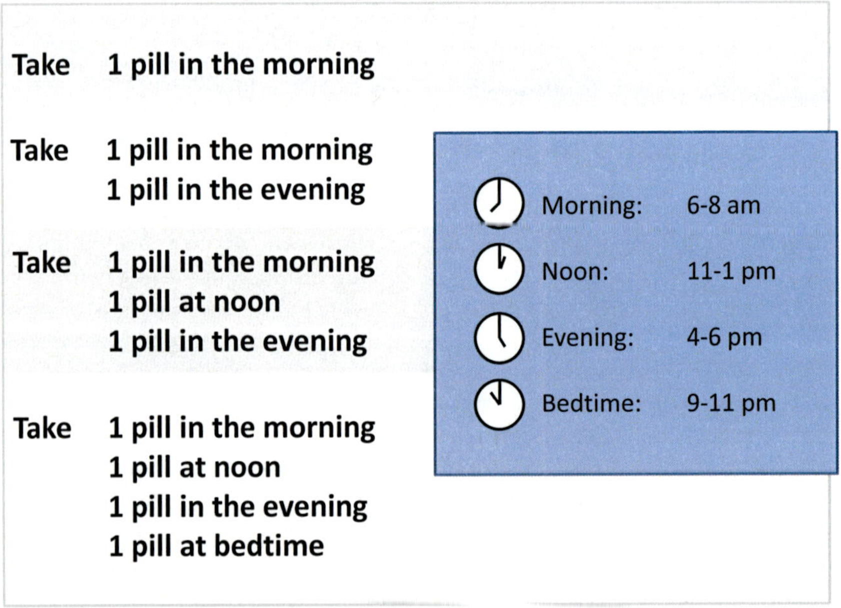

FIGURE 5-2 An example of a Universal Medication Schedule.
SOURCE: As presented by Michael Wolf, November 16, 2017.

does not mean that we should not be doing it." What he and his colleagues have found, though, is that any health literacy intervention, whether it is on auxiliary warning labels, prescription dosing instructions, or medication guides, does improve outcome significantly across all levels of health literacy (Sahm et al., 2012; Wolf et al., 2010, 2011, 2014). "The disparity between the highest functioning literate patients and those with the lowest literacy skills does not shrink," Wolf explained. "You are not going to get the benefit you need using written materials if you cannot read very well. It just makes sense."

Another takeaway from the accumulated body of evidence is that variable content for prescription medications still exists. "We need to get past this," said Wolf. "It is just an amazing thing that we cannot find a way to have standardized content about what needs to be known about a particular medication because then we can start having the conversation about how to improve it and then how best to disseminate it." The fact that educational materials vary so dramatically, he added, is a major hindrance to moving forward with evidence-based interventions. In addition, despite a decade of work stressing the importance of the relationship between provider and patient, spoken counseling from physicians, nurses, and pharmacists remains infrequent and inadequate. Multifaceted communications strategies that engage providers and that are co-developed with patients are needed to make truly meaningful changes in how patients learn about and use their medications, said Wolf.

Moving forward, Wolf said the field needs to set standards that go beyond written materials. He acknowledged that USP has done a good job establishing and promoting standards for written materials. Now is the time to look closely at how those standards translate into how the field develops, designs, and disseminates digital tools that communicate information and support patients' behaviors with their medications, he said. He noted there is an expansive literature that identifies ways to optimize written health materials (Jacobson and Parker, 2014) as well as evidence on how to design robust multimedia materials (Mayer, 2005). There is even a tool that AHRQ created, the Patient Education Materials Assessment Tool (PEMAT),[4] that those who develop materials can use to assess understandability and actionability. However, he added, despite this body of literature and tools such as PEMAT, recommended principles are ignored more often than not.

Commenting on how he wishes the discussion could move beyond what font size to use when creating written materials, Wolf said that bridging the many divides is going to be very challenging going forward given how the system of health care delivery in the United States is "one of our great-

[4] See http://www.ahrq.gov/professionals/prevention-chronic-care/improve/self-mgmt/pemat/index.html (accessed March 31, 2017).

est adversaries in terms of trying to give people good information about their medicines." Today, for example, even coordinating communications between the pharmacist and physician is difficult, and interventions aimed at addressing that problem have not had much success. The lack of interoperability among electronic health records (EHRs) and pharmacy labeling systems exacerbates this problem, said Wolf. Except for the rare health system with embedded pharmacies, it is difficult to create interventions in which the physician at the prescribing end and pharmacist at the dispensing end can reinforce each other's messages and provide adequate counseling to patients.

Part of the solution, he proposed, is that the EHR might serve as the focal point for such coordination. In fact, he and his colleagues are working in partnership with Walgreens and UnitedHealthcare to examine how it may be possible to leverage technology to allow pharmacists to provide extensive support to patients, with the key being that pharmacists will need to have access to a patient's medication list and their EHR.

Moving beyond written information, Wolf mentioned a recent paper that reviewed 16 trials targeting medication adherence using mobile phone text reminders (Thakkar et al., 2016). A meta-analysis of these 16 studies showed that a simple ongoing text reminder service produced an average two-fold increase in medication adherence. He said that while many technology platforms might have the potential to improve medication adherence and safety, most are not matched to patient needs, and these modalities may not match patient preferences. In 2014, he and his colleagues surveyed user reviews of the approximately 400 mobile phone apps for medication self-management and found that their design was largely not patient centered (Bailey et al., 2014). In fact, he said, few of these apps were designed with input from patients and so perhaps it is not surprising they do not address the barriers patients face in using their medications properly.

Wolf concluded his presentation with a brief discussion of a system he and his collaborators on working on with Eli Lilly and Company that can use the EHR to create multiple points of providing information to patients about their medications (see Figure 5-3). For example, this system would use the EHR to prompt physicians with best practice alerts when they write a prescription and provide counseling advice on what they can say to their patients. The system would also automatically generate a one-page medication guide summary that would include a link to the medication order and an after-visit summary. The patient would receive automated prompts via email or phone that would ask them to use their patient portal to report on how they are doing with medication, if they are having problems, if they have missed any doses, or if they have experienced any side effects. The system would also generate an EHR care alert for any patient at risk as determined by that medication check.

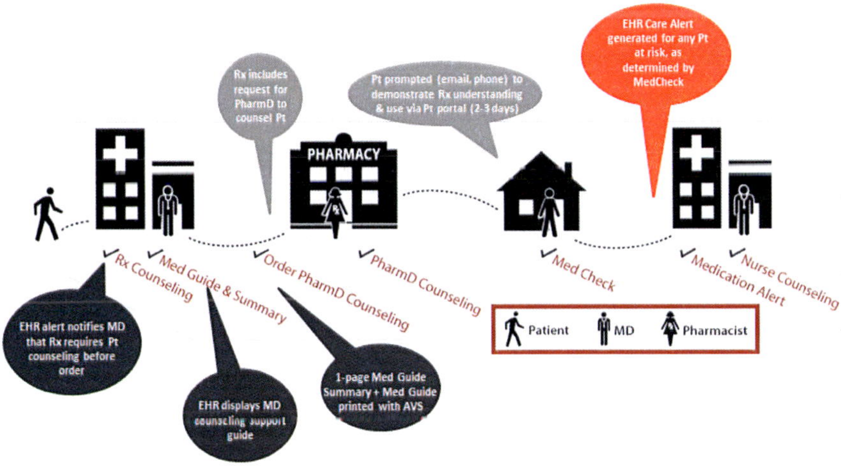

FIGURE 5-3 An electronic health record–based system that would provide multiple opportunities for providing patients with medication information and assistance.
NOTE: AVS = after visit summary; EHR = electronic health record; MD = medical doctor; PharmD = doctor of pharmacy; Pt = patient; Rx = prescription.
SOURCE: As presented by Michael Wolf, November 17, 2016.

In closing, Wolf said there are many good interventions and innovations available, as well as some that are horrible, but the important point is to test these interventions and use the ones supported by evidence. "We need to get out of the way of ourselves and just start doing something, to know that we can evaluate it and if it does not work, we can learn something from it," said Wolf. "I do not think we are going to be doing something worse than what we are already doing right now."

DISCUSSION

Brach opened the discussion by asking Rennie to clarify how manufacturers can rewrite and change FDA-approved labeling to reflect focus group assessments given that FDA-approved language is sacrosanct. Rennie replied that the testing and revision process happens before the sponsor submits labeling language to FDA. The testing and revision process is built into the time line that her company, and she supposed every other pharmaceutical company, develops for the drug approval process, and it starts well before FDA is ready to grant approval for a new medication.

Marin Allen from the National Institutes of Health commented on the need for the manufacturer of a drug, who knows more about it than anyone, to share responsibility with physicians to ensure that patients understand how best to take their medications. In her opinion, the onus for doing so should not rest solely with physicians. She also remarked that patients are being confused by the disclaimer messages that accompany television drug advertising, which she said she understands fulfills a legal requirement, but does little to tell patients what a given medication will do for them. Rennie responded to Marin's call for the pharmaceutical industry to try to address these two concerns by noting that those very concerns drive Merck's efforts to make health literacy a requirement. "We do think that the physician's time is limited and not everyone out there has an incentive to educate the patients, and so when we have a new product coming on board, and for the products that we do have, we take that role seriously," said Rennie. "We all want to do what's in the best interest for patients, and certainly from a legal perspective, I want to make sure that patients have all the information that they need to take the product safely."

Rosof asked the panelists to comment on what they believe would be valuable to the roundtable in thinking about health-literate design going forward, and in doing so, to be innovative. Morrow replied that he thinks it important to help people not only find information, but also evaluate and integrate information across multiple documents in an online environment. "We know, at least anecdotally, that people are being nudged all the time by the way websites are designed to go elsewhere, and they may not remember to come back," he said. A useful step, he noted, may be to think about this problem in terms of the way animals forage for food, where they are constantly adapting to the ecosystem in terms of where to look. In that respect, there are theories of information foraging that can help people evaluate information and make on-the-fly assessments about whether they have got the information they needed to answer their questions or if they need to continue their search elsewhere. Such theories may be particularly useful for helping older adults who spend too much time reading text online, whereas younger adults tend to be better information foragers and are better able to remember more information across multiple information sources. "I think there is interesting work in computer science that embraces the idea of ecology of information and how it is transforming with the new media," said Morrow.

Rennie said she has observed over the past decade that there has been a move to put more information into patient medication guides and physician prescribing information. "That has had the effect of making patients overwhelmed, quite frankly," said Rennie. Instead of listing every possible side effect, perhaps a better way to go would be to list the most common ones and then include a statement as simple as "If anything changes, make sure you call your doctor because it could be a side effect." In her opinion, that type of discrimination among which side effects to list would go a long way toward helping patients and alerting them to pay attention to how they react when taking a prescription drug. She also commented on the message she heard that the pharmaceutical industry does not do a good enough job telling patients why it is important for them to take their medications. "It used to be that pharmaceutical companies did more of that," she said, noting that companies do less of that now in response to warning letters from FDA regarding the need to have outcomes data to be able to discuss outcomes of the disease. "I think we need to figure out how we can fill that void to let patients know not only here is the condition, but why it is critically important if their physician has prescribed this medication to take it so that you can hopefully stave off this sort of bad outcomes in the future," said Rennie.

Giving context to his comments, Wolf said what he cares about is helping patients get the optimal benefit of the medications they are prescribed, to be able to take them, minimize any harm associated with them, and also be properly vigilant so they can problem solve and seek care if necessary. From that perspective, he said many things can help patients, such as disseminating good content through patient portals, but implementing these types of interventions means overcoming barriers by engaging more with providers. "Whether that is a care coordinator, a pharmacist, or an allied health care provider, we need some way to have ongoing relations with patients between encounters, and maybe even start by focusing on those who are at greatest risk, such as those patients who have a lot of medications to take," said Wolf. That is where he hopes the roundtable can be creative in thinking about how health care is being redesigned and how to create more linkages for knowledge exchange in a health-literate manner that engages patients in their own care and supports behaviors that encourage them to seek information and problem solve about their medications.

Jennifer Dillaha with the Arkansas Department of Health commented that the growing number of older adults who are not likely to improve their own health literacy skills places a burden on an increasing number of families to gain the skills needed to understand proper medication use. She asked Morrow if the Internet work his group has conducted could be applied to patient portals, which is where many family members and other caregivers will go to get the information they need. Morrow replied that he has a project under way that is being driven, in part, by his frustration about using his patient portal to understand clinical test results. "It is abundantly clear that the best practices that we have been talking about today are not being used routinely in terms of designing the information that is on patient portals," said Morrow. This project is attempting to present information in a way that will enable older adults to understand the risk implications of the numeric information from test results, such as cholesterol and triglyceride levels. Relying heavily on graphical representations, he and his team are moving toward developing a conversational agent interface that would provide an interaction with a virtual physician who can provide high-level commentary on the accompanying graphics. "The idea is not to do an end run around face-to-face communication with your doctor, but to help bridge that gap," said Morrow. In some respects, he added, this type of system would provide patient decision support in the way that an EHR can provide clinical decision support to the physician.

Catina O'Leary from Health Literacy Media noted that despite all of the good interventions that have been developed, nothing seems to disrupt the system in a way that enables those interventions to gain much of a foothold and then spread in the nation's health care systems. Wolf agreed with that assessment and said that like O'Leary, he is tired of coming to meetings and hearing the same things that he has been hearing for the past 15 years. "I am sick of going to multiple meetings at different agencies and feeling like I am having the same conversation over again," said Wolf. He added that his frustration over the lack of progress is one reason why he and his colleagues are working to use the EHR as the focus of a system that will automatically alert physicians about the need to provide more information to patients about their medications and to provide that information in plain language the physician can use.

One component of this system that he is working on now is a way of tracking how often physicians provide the necessary information and creating a metric that could serve as a quality indicator and give feedback to the physician. Wolf added, though, that patients need to be accountable, too, particularly those who are taking multiple medications. Physicians could ask patients to check into their portals every few weeks and report on how they are doing with their medications by answering a short questionnaire, for example.

James Duhig from AbbVie Inc. noted that his company has a program for one of its major products that has several hundred nurses trained in cultural competencies who can provide health-literate information on this product. The challenge, he said, is to reproduce that type of support system for products that do not generate billions of dollars in revenue. He then asked if the goal of the health literacy community is to continue being an add-on, or if the goal is to make health literacy an integral component of medication outcomes. Wolf said he is encouraged by the way in which health literacy is now seen as part of appreciating the user experience and that the field is starting to benefit from human factors research, cognitive psychology, and efforts to design learning environments.

In Wolf's opinion, the health literacy field needs to make sure that in this time of a growing emphasis on patient engagement that health literacy is at the table for those conversations. Health literacy, he said, needs to become active in organizations such as the American Public Health Association, the Society of General Internal Medicine, and AcademyHealth, and to have representation in the special interest groups advocating for more patient engagement. The health literacy field needs to do a better job conveying that health literacy is more than just putting complex ideas into plan language. "We are a behavioral science, not just an information science," said Wolf. In his opinion, health literacy needs to be seen as a field focused on using information better to engage patients to make them care more about their own health.

Morrow said Wolf's comments reminded him of the discussions that used to be held about how to infuse human factors into organizations so that they are "breathing the concept" and that it becomes an embedded competency. FDA, he said, has led the charge on this front, and human factors is gradually becoming an inherent part of the process at many organizations. He noted that achieving the same status for health literacy would be helped by the ongoing work on health-literate organizations and how they function. Rennie added that one important area in which health literacy needs to become an integral part of the design process is in the social media world given the central role social media plays for younger adults when they look for information on what might be ailing them. "They do not call a health care provider, they go onto Google and try to figure it out," said Rennie. It is imperative, then, to determine how to help ensure that people going to social media and the Internet for information are getting accurate, complete, and not misleading information. The industry has not yet figured out the best way to use social media, she concluded.

6

Reflections on the Day

Cindy Brach began the traditional Roundtable on Health Literacy practice of providing the members' thoughts on the day's presentations and discussions by noting that what she took away from the patient panel was the need for more shared decision making in medication decisions and understanding the lived experiences that must be incorporated in those decisions. Caleb Sexton expressed the need for empathy, Bobbie Reed spoke of her frustrations at having her ideas about her son's medications summarily dismissed by her son's physicians, and both Reed and Darvece Monson pointed to the importance of presenting information at the right time, when an individual is not at a cognitive low point and unable to absorb and understand information. These comments, she said, led her to wonder if there are options akin to nurse advice lines that could be an accountable place for patients and caregivers to go to get answers when they are ready to hear information or if they have questions they need answered after throwing away the materials the pharmacist handed them with their prescription.

Another message from the first panel that Brach highlighted was the importance of the care team and the need to make better use of all-care team members as sources of information. She raised the idea of requiring counseling at the time of dispensing, which is what Canada does, and wondered what roles team members could play that would result in patients and caregivers having a better understanding of their medication regimens. Brach's final comment was that perhaps the roundtable could help get the message to electronic health record vendors and the companies that create pharmacy labeling systems about the need to make information more accessible, understandable, and actionable.

Jane Grover said her main impression from the workshop was that there is an opportunity to not only integrate between the medical and dental worlds, but to bring health literacy into the world of dentistry. There is, she noted, an advisory committee on health literacy in dentistry, but dentistry is typically not team based. She pointed out that every patient has a mouth, and there is an opportunity to bring health literacy to oral health concepts into dentistry,

Lori Hall said that though she has been a roundtable member for 3 years, it was only since January 2016 that she was given the title of director of health literacy at Eli Lilly and Company. She credited her roundtable colleague Laurie Myers of Merck with blazing the trail for having dedicated health literacy teams in pharmaceutical companies. She then noted that the organization's seriousness about health literacy started to change when she was given that official title, so she recommended that others doing health literacy work in pharmaceutical companies should advocate for a job title that has "health literacy" in it. For her, the impact of getting that title is that she has since received 139 unsolicited requests for input from every point along the drug development continuum at Merck. This is important, she said, because, "What I am hearing over and over again today is the further upstream we can apply health literacy in the research, clinical research, and the approval and commercialization of medications, all patients benefit." She then invited all pharmaceutical companies to join this non-competitive effort. Kim Parson from Humana also supported the idea of introducing health literacy concepts as early in the research and development process as possible and noted the importance of bringing the consumers of medications into the design process as early as possible.

Jennifer Dillaha said it was clear to her how much work needs to be done to help people understand the information available to them on medication and other health-related topics. In particular, commenting on Heather Rennie's remarks about the need to help patients and caregivers distinguish between factual and misleading, non-factual information, she said the field is going to need to work on that aspect of information gathering as an important piece of the health literacy skill set.

Wilma Alvarado-Little said she appreciated the comments of the day's first panel because they highlighted the importance of empowering vulnerable populations and the need to meet patients where they are to address their concerns. "They are the experts about themselves and they are not given the voice in the room to be told it is okay to ask that question or to say something like, 'This is too much information,'" said Alvarado-Little. She noted how she appreciates when her providers can acknowledge they do not know the answer to one of her questions because that is actually a very sophisticated response and it means the provider is listening to her.

Myers said pharmaceutical companies need to address many things besides patient labeling in terms of health literacy. Clinical trials materials, for example, need to be understandable by people with low health literacy, and in particular, among individuals of underrepresented populations. Her concern is that while there are efforts to include patient perspectives in clinical trials, only the most articulate patients are part of that process today. Informed consent is another area that needs more attention from a health literacy perspective, as is the development of instructions of use for combination products. Myers also thought it is imperative to understand the met and unmet needs of patients who desire future products in terms of patient-reported outcomes and other quality measures. "Thinking about consumerism, how do we demonstrate the value of our products to patients? What are the quality measures that are important to them?" she asked.

Steven Rush from UnitedHealth Group said he had a mixed reaction to the workshop. On the one hand, as others had mentioned, he was disappointed to hear many of the same issues raised that he has been hearing for many years. At the same time, he did hear of some progress and is encouraged by the resources and approaches being brought to bear on the challenge of helping patients understand their medications. "Maybe they are not big changes, but there are changes, so that has been exciting," said Rush. He noted that the concept of cognitive burden resonated with him because it makes real comments he hears from patients about having to think too much about their medications.

For Jay Duhig, the discussions at the workshop left him "incredibly hopeful." Underlying that sense of optimism were the presentations by the members of the first panel, who were so articulate about their experiences and what is meaningful with regard to their care; the inclusion of the many stakeholders that need to be engaged in the effort to communicate more clearly about medications; and by the case studies of data-driven, outcome-driven interventions presented in the afternoon session.

Michael Villaire from the Institute for Healthcare Advancement agreed with the previous comments that the first panel was a highlight of the workshop and he thanked the panelists for sharing their stories and struggles. He commented that efforts to redesign systems are needed and are a critical part of what the health literacy community does. Medications, however, are still personal, taken by individuals, not systems, and not taken for a variety of personal reasons that need to be acknowledged and accepted. While systems-based approaches can address the large majority of issues, they will not fix every issue for every person. "That one-on-one interaction between individuals from the health care system and people who are trying to access the health care system is really the critical juncture, and, frankly, it is where we spend the least amount of time in the entire health care system," said Villaire. "My recommendation is to incentivize those interactions, extend that amount of time, use other providers, navigators, and educators, but to provide them when they are needed by the patient." He also suggested that the pharmacy could provide a place where patients can receive help in a shame-free and cost-free environment.

Bernard Rosof noted that he is "not uncomfortable with hearing things over and over and over again until we get it right." In fact, he added, "that is the principle of quality improvement and performance improvement, and that is to be transparent and say it again and again and again until you do get it right." He then read an email with comments from Robert Logan, who wrote that in his opinion it would be good to embed a health literacy perspective as part of the future postmarketing surveillance initiatives. Logan noted that Will Shrank told the workshop that the U.S. Food and Drug Administration's (FDA's) postmarketing surveillance efforts are primarily epidemiological and overlook the social determinants of health that impact medication adherence, safety, and administration. He also recalled that in May 2017, he heard FDA Commissioner Robert Califf suggest that postmarketing surveillance efforts may be insufficiently multidimensional to address contemporary drug safety-related issues and may need to be expanded. "I envision an important role for the roundtable to gather evidence and provide guidance about how to embed a health literacy perspective as part of revamped postmarketing surveillance initiatives," wrote Logan. "A health literacy perspective would enrich data collection for medication safety, efficacy, and administration."

Linda Harris from the U.S. Department of Health and Human Services (HHS) started her comments by introducing Lee Zwanziger, the newly appointed co-chair of the HHS working group on health literacy. She said she appreciated that the workshop included presentations on user-centered design and Dan Morrow's presentation on interdisciplinary skills. She noted the importance of including work on cognitive challenges affecting executive function, given the role that executive function plays in the ability to read and problem solve. "We need to be bringing that science into the way we are thinking about health literacy because it is so much more than just reading."

Before adjourning the workshop, Rosof asked the workshop participants to take a moment and remember Margaret Loveland, who passed away on August 26, 2016. Loveland was a former member of the roundtable and long-time supporter of health literacy in her leadership role at Merck. "Always a valuable and loved member of the roundtable, her analytic input, her insights, and her ability to contribute to what we have accomplished over the past decade or so has been on everybody's mind," said Rosof.

References

AHRQ (Agency for Healthcare Research and Quality). 2014. *AHRQ pharmacy health literacy center.* http://www.ahrq.gov/professionals/quality-patient-safety/pharmhealthlit/index.html (accessed December 5, 2016).

Bailey, S. C., L. T. Belter, A. U. Pandit, D. M. Carpenter, E. Carlos, and M. S. Wolf. 2014. The availability, functionality, and quality of mobile applications supporting medication self-management. *Journal of the American Medical Informatics Association* 21(3):542-546.

Bailey, S. C., P. Navaratnam, H. Black, A. L. Russell, and M. S. Wolf. 2015. Advancing best practices for prescription drug labeling. *Annals of Pharmacotherapy* 49(11):1222-1236.

Bates, D. W., D. J. Cullen, N. Laird, L. A. Petersen, S. D. Small, D. Servi, G. Laffel, B. J. Sweitzer, B. F. Shea, R. Hallisey, et al. 1995. Incidence of adverse drug events and potential adverse drug events. Implications for prevention. ADE prevention study group. *JAMA* 274(1):29-34.

Budnitz, D. S., and P. M. Layde. 2007. Outpatient drug safety: New steps in an old direction. *Pharmacoepidemiology and Drug Safety* 16(2):160-165.

Cancino, R. S., L. Culpepper, E. Sadikova, J. Martin, B. W. Jack, and S. E. Mitchell. 2014. Dose–response relationship between depressive symptoms and hospital readmission. *Journal of Hospital Medicine* 9(6):358-364.

CDER (Center for Drug Evaluation and Research). 2013. *Guidance for industry: Safety considerations for container labels and carton labeling design to minimize medication errors.* Rockville, MD: U.S. Food and Drug Administration.

CDER. 2016. *Human factors studies and related clinical study considerations in combination product design and development; draft guidance for industry and Food and Drug Administration staff; availability.*

Chin, J., D. G. Morrow, E. A. Stine-Morrow, T. Conner-Garcia, J. F. Graumlich, and M. D. Murray. 2011. The process-knowledge model of health literacy: Evidence from a componential analysis of two commonly used measures. *Journal of Health Communication* 16(Suppl 3):222-241.

Chin, J., A. Madison, X. Gao, J. F. Graumlich, T. Conner-Garcia, M. D. Murray, E. A. Stine-Morrow, and D. G. Morrow. 2015. Cognition and health literacy in older adults' recall of self-care information. *Gerontologist* 57(2):261-268.

Czaja, S. J., J. Sharit, C. C. Lee, S. N. Nair, M. A. Hernandez, N. Arana, and S. H. Fu. 2013. Factors influencing use of an e-health website in a community sample of older adults. *Journal of the American Medical Informatics Association* 20(2):277-284.

Davis, T. C., M. S. Wolf, P. F. Bass, 3rd, M. Middlebrooks, E. Kennen, D. W. Baker, C. L. Bennett, R. Durazo-Arvizu, A. Bocchini, S. Savory, and R. M. Parker. 2006a. Low literacy impairs comprehension of prescription drug warning labels. *Journal of General Internal Medicine* 21(8):847-851.

Davis, T. C., M. S. Wolf, P. F. Bass, 3rd, J. A. Thompson, H. H. Tilson, M. Neuberger, and R. M. Parker. 2006b. Literacy and misunderstanding prescription drug labels. *Annals of Internal Medicine* 145(12):887-894.

Fialová, D., and G. Onder. 2009. Medication errors in elderly people: Contributing factors and future perspectives. *British Journal of Clinical Pharmacology* 67(6):641-645.

Halpern, S. D., B. French, D. S. Small, K. Saulsgiver, M. O. Harhay, J. Audrain-McGovern, G. Loewenstein, T. A. Brennan, D. A. Asch, and K. G. Volpp. 2015. Randomized trial of four financial-incentive programs for smoking cessation. *New England Journal of Medicine* 372(22):2108-2117.

IOM (Institute of Medicine). 2000. *To err is human: Building a safer health system.* Washington, DC: National Academy Press.

IOM. 2001. *Crossing the quality chasm: A new health system for the 21st century*. Washington, DC: National Academy Press.

IOM. 2007. *Preventing medication errors: Quality chasm series.* Washington, DC: The National Academies Press.

IOM. 2008. *Standardizing medication labels: Confusing patients less: Workshop summary.* Washington, DC: The National Academies Press.

Jack, B., J. Greenwald, S. Forsythe, J. O'Donnell, A. Johnson, L. Schipelliti, M. Goodwin, G. Burniske, C. Hesko, M. Paasche-Orlow, C. Manasseh, D. Anthony, S. Martin, L. Hollister, M. Jack, V. Jhaveri, K. Casey, and V. K. Chetty. 2008. Developing the tools to administer a comprehensive hospital discharge program: The reengineered discharge (RED) program. In *Advances in patient safety: New directions and alternative approaches: performance and tools. AHRQ Pub. No. 08-0034-3.* Vol. 3, edited by Henriksen K., J. B. Battles, M. A. Keyes, and M. L. Grady. Rockville, MD: Agency for Healthcare Research and Quality.

Jack, B. W., V. K. Chetty, D. Anthony, J. L. Greenwald, G. M. Sanchez, A. E. Johnson, S. R. Forsythe, J. K. O'Donnell, M. K. Paasche-Orlow, C. Manasseh, S. Martin, and L. Culpepper. 2009. A reengineered hospital discharge program to decrease rehospitalization: A randomized trial. *Annals of Internal Medicine* 150(3):178-187.

Jacobson, K. L., and R. M. Parker. 2014. *Health literacy principles guidance for making information understandable, useful, and navigable.* Discussion Paper edited by Institute of Medicine. Washington, DC: The National Academies Press.

Koper, D., G. Kamenski, M. Flamm, B. Bohmdorfer, and A. Sonnichsen. 2013. Frequency of medication errors in primary care patients with polypharmacy. *Family Practice* 30(3): 313-319.

Mayer, M. 2005. *The Cambridge handbook of multimedia learning*. Cambridge, UK: Cambridge University Press.

Mitchell, S. E., M. K. Paasche-Orlow, S. R. Forsythe, V. K. Chetty, J. K. O'Donnell, J. L. Greenwald, L. Culpepper, and B. W. Jack. 2010. Post-discharge hospital utilization among adult medical inpatients with depressive symptoms. *Journal of Hospital Medicine* 5(7):378-384.

Mitchell, S. E., E. Sadikova, B. W. Jack, and M. K. Paasche-Orlow. 2012. Health literacy and 30-day post-discharge hospital utilization. *Journal of Health Communication* 17(Suppl 3):325-338.

Mitchell, S. E., P. M. Gardiner, E. Sadikova, J. M. Martin, B. W. Jack, J. H. Hibbard, and M. K. Paasche-Orlow. 2014. Patient activation and 30-day post-discharge hospital utilization. *Journal of General Internal Medicine* 29(2):349-355.

NCPIE (National Council on Patient Information and Education). 2013. *Accelerating progress in prescription medication adherence: The adherence action agenda. A national action plan to address America's "other drug problem."* Rockville, MD: NCPIE.

NQF (National Quality Forum). 2006. *Safe practices for better healthcare 2006 update: A consensus report.* Washington, DC: National Quality Forum.

NQF. 2010. *Safe practices for better healthcare 2010 update: A consensus report.* Washington, DC: National Quality Forum.

Persell, S. D., C. Y. Osborn, R. Richard, S. Skripkauskas, and M. S. Wolf. 2007. Limited health literacy is a barrier to medication reconciliation in ambulatory care. *Journal of General Internal Medicine* 22(11):1523-1526.

Sahm, L. J., M. S. Wolf, L. M. Curtis, R. Behan, M. Brennan, H. Gallwey, and S. McCarthy. 2012. What's in a label? An exploratory study of patient-centered drug instructions. *European Journal of Clinical Pharmacology* 68(5):777-782.

Sarkar, U., A. Lopez, J. H. Maselli, and R. Gonzales. 2011. Adverse drug events in U.S. adult ambulatory medical care. *Health Services Research* 46(5):1517-1533.

Sharit, J., M. A. Hernandez, S. J. Czaja, and P. Pirolli. 2008. Investigating the roles of knowledge and cognitive abilities in older adult information seeking on the web. *ACM Transactions on Computer-Human Interaction* 15(1):3.

Shrank, W., J. Avorn, C. Rolon, and P. Shekelle. 2007. Effect of content and format of prescription drug labels on readability, understanding, and medication use: A systematic review. *Annals of Pharmacotherapy* 41(5):783-801.

Shrank, W. H., R. M. Parker, T. C. Davis, A. U. Pandit, J. P. Knox, P. Moraras, A. Rademaker, and M. S. Wolf. 2010. Rationale and design of a randomized trial to evaluate an evidence-based prescription drug label on actual medication use. *Contemporary Clinical Trials* 31(6):564-571.

Taha, J., S. J. Czaja, J. Sharit, and D. G. Morrow. 2013. Factors affecting usage of a personal health record (PHR) to manage health. *Psychology and Aging* 28(4):1124-1139.

Taha, J., J. Sharit, and S. J. Czaja. 2014. The impact of numeracy ability and technology skills on older adults' performance of health management tasks using a patient portal. *Journal of Applied Gerontology* 33(4):416-436.

Tarn, D. M., J. Heritage, D. A. Paterniti, R. D. Hays, R. L. Kravitz, and N. S. Wenger. 2006. Physician communication when prescribing new medications. *Archives of Internal Medicine* 166(17):1855-1862.

Tarn, D. M., D. A. Paterniti, D. K. Orosz, C. H. Tseng, and N. S. Wenger. 2013. Intervention to enhance communication about newly prescribed medications. *Annals of Family Medicine* 11(1):28-36.

Thakkar, J., R. Kurup, T. L. Laba, K. Santo, A. Thiagalingam, A. Rodgers, M. Woodward, J. Redfern, and C. K. Chow. 2016. Mobile telephone text messaging for medication adherence in chronic disease: A meta-analysis. *JAMA Internal Medicine* 176(3):340-349.

Vrijens, B., S. De Geest, D. A. Hughes, K. Przemyslaw, J. Demonceau, T. Ruppar, F. Dobbels, E. Fargher, V. Morrison, P. Lewek, M. Matyjaszczyk, C. Mshelia, W. Clyne, J. K. Aronson, and J. Urquhart. 2012. A new taxonomy for describing and defining adherence to medications. *British Journal of Clinical Pharmacology* 73(5):691-705.

Wali, H., Z. Hudani, S. Wali, K. Mercer, and K. Grindrod. 2016. A systematic review of interventions to improve medication information for low health literate populations. *Research in Social & Administrative Pharmacy* 12(6):830-864.

Wolf, M. S., T. C. Davis, H. H. Tilson, P. F. Bass, 3rd, and R. M. Parker. 2006. Misunderstanding of prescription drug warning labels among patients with low literacy. *American Journal of Health-System Pharmacy* 63(11):1048-1055.

Wolf, M. S., T. C. Davis, P. F. Bass, L. M. Curtis, L. A. Lindquist, J. A. Webb, M. V. Bocchini, S. C. Bailey, and R. M. Parker. 2010. Improving prescription drug warnings to promote patient comprehension. *Archives of Internal Medicine* 170(1):50-56.

Wolf, M. S., T. C. Davis, L. M. Curtis, J. A. Webb, S. C. Bailey, W. H. Shrank, L. Lindquist, B. Ruo, M. V. Bocchini, R. M. Parker, and A. J. Wood. 2011. Effect of standardized, patient-centered label instructions to improve comprehension of prescription drug use. *Medical Care* 49(1):96-100.

Wolf, M. S., S. C. Bailey, M. Serper, M. Smith, T. C. Davis, A. L. Russell, B. S. Manzoor, L. Belter, R. M. Parker, and B. Lambert. 2014. Comparative effectiveness of patient-centered strategies to improve FDA medication guides. *Medical Care* 52(9):781-789.

Wolf, M. S., T. C. Davis, L. M. Curtis, S. C. Bailey, J. P. Knox, A. Bergeron, M. Abbet, W. H. Shrank, R. M. Parker, and A. J. Wood. 2016. A patient-centered prescription drug label to promote appropriate medication use and adherence. *Journal of General Internal Medicine* 31(12):1482-1489.

Appendix A

Workshop Agenda

Roundtable on Health Literacy
The National Academies of Sciences, Engineering, and Medicine
NAS 120
2101 Constitution Avenue, NW
Washington, DC 20418

Communicating Clearly About Medicine: A Workshop
November 17, 2016
Agenda

Workshop Objective:

The workshop seeks to address the question, "How do we provide clear written communications to patients?" with a focus on the patient experience.

8:30-8:45 **Welcome and Workshop Overview**
Bernard Rosof, M.D., MACP
Chair, Roundtable on Health Literacy

8:45-9:30 **The Patient Experience**
Darvece A. Monson, patient and advocate
Caleb Sexton, patient and advocate
Bobbie Reed, caregiver and advocate
Moderator: Terri Ann Parnell, D.N.P., RN

9:30-10:00 **Discussion**

10:00-10:15 BREAK

10:15-10:20 **Introductions**

10:20-10:40 **Current Landscape of Research on Written Communications**
Will Shrank, M.D., M.S.H.S.
Chief Medical Officer
University of Pittsburgh Medical Center Health Plan

10:40-11:00 **The Role of Human Factors Engineering**
Irene Chan, Pharm.D., BCPS
Division of Medication Error Prevention and Analysis
Office of Surveillance and Epidemiology
U.S. Food and Drug Administration

Elisabeth Walther, Pharm.D., J.D.
Division of Medical Policy Programs
Office of Medical Policy
U.S. Food and Drug Administration

11:00-11:20 **Human-Centered Design**
Ed Israelski, Ph.D.
Consultant, Technical Advisor on Human Factors
Retired Director, Human Factors
AbbVie Inc.

11:20-12:00 **Discussion**

12:00-1:00 LUNCH

Translating Research into Practice Case Studies

1:00-1:05 **Introductions**

1:05-1:20 **Adopting an Easy-to-Read Medication Label in Wisconsin**
Steve Sparks, M.S.
Health Literacy Director
Wisconsin Health Literacy

1:20-1:35 **Including Individuals with Low Health Literacy in Research and Development of New Labeling**
Laurie Myers, M.B.A.
Global Health Literacy Director
Merck Sharp & Dohme Corp.

1:35-1:50	**Project RED: Engaging Patients in Medication Management at Hospital Discharge** *Brian Jack, M.D.* *Professor and Chair, Department of Family Medicine* *Boston University School of Medicine*
1:50-2:05	**Planning for Non-English–Speaking Patients** *Charles Lee, M.D.* *President and Founder* *Polyglot Systems*
2:05-2:25	**Reactor Panel** *Donna Horn, R.Ph., D.Ph.* *Director, Patient Safety, Community Pharmacy* *Institute for Safe Medication Practices* *H. Shonna Yin, M.D., M.S.* *Associate Professor of Pediatrics and Population Health* *Departments of Pediatrics and Population Health* *New York University School of Medicine/ Bellevue Hospital Center*
2:25-3:00	**Discussion**
3:00-3:15	BREAK

The Future of Health-Literate Design

3:15-3:20	**Introductions**
3:20-3:35	**Written Materials in the Digital Space** *Dan Morrow, Ph.D.* *Chair, Department of Educational Psychology,* *University of Illinois at Urbana-Champaign*
3:35-3:50	**Legal Considerations in Applying Health Literacy Principles to Written Communications** *Heather Rennie, J.D.* *Managing Counsel, Regulatory Legal Group* *Merck Sharp & Dohme Corp.*

3:50-4:10 **Moving Forward in Written Communications Research**
Mike Wolf, Ph.D.
Professor, Medicine and Learning Sciences
Associate Division Chief, Research
Division of General Internal Medicine
Feinberg School of Medicine
Northwestern University

4:10-4:45 **Discussion**

4:45-5:30 **Reflections on the Day**

5:30 ADJOURN

Appendix B

Biographical Sketches of Workshop Speakers, Moderators, and Reactors

Irene Z. Chan, Pharm.D., received a B.S. in pharmacy and doctor of pharmacy degree from Rutgers University Ernest Mario School of Pharmacy. After graduation she was called to active duty by the U.S. Public Health Service and assigned to the Gallup Indian Medical Center in Gallup, New Mexico, an Indian Health Service (IHS) facility, where she completed a postgraduate year 1 pharmacy practice residency. After completing her residency, she worked with the IHS for more than 5 years in Gallup and Santa Fe, in both inpatient and outpatient pharmacy settings. During her time with IHS, her responsibilities included chairing a multidisciplinary medication safety task force, serving as supervisor of inpatient pharmacy services, and serving as the pharmacy residency program director. While stationed in New Mexico, Commander (CDR) Chan also worked closely with the New Mexico Pharmacists Association, serving in various leadership positions within the state association. In 2009, CDR Chan transferred to the U.S. Food and Drug Administration, where she serves as deputy director in the Division of Medication Error Prevention and Analysis, responsible for leveraging her knowledge of regulatory science, human factors, and risk management to provide oversight of safety recommendations regarding drug nomenclature, labels, labeling, packaging, and product design.

Donna Horn, R.Ph., D.Ph., directs the Institute for Safe Medication Practices' (ISMP's) patient safety activities in community/ambulatory practice. Dr. Horn serves as an author and editor of ISMP's four newsletters for acute care providers, nurses, ambulatory/community care providers, and consumers. She has more than 25 years of experience in the retail/chain community pharmacy practice setting, as the privacy officer and manager of regulatory affairs for Brooks/Eckerd Pharmacy, where she wrote numerous policies and procedures to govern pharmacists working in chain pharmacy and as a pharmacist and regional pharmacy manager for Osco Drug. Prior to joining ISMP, she served as president and chair of the National Association of Boards of Pharmacy, where her focus was on patient safety, primarily on reducing medication errors in community pharmacy. Dr. Horn also served 11 years on the Massachusetts Board of Registration in Pharmacy as both a member and as president. Her work has focused on continuous quality improvement, policies on promoting ease of access to appropriate reference materials, monitoring prescription usage in chronic disease state patients, drug recall procedures, proper staffing guidelines, and incorporating strategies to optimize therapeutic outcomes. Most recently Dr. Horn was elected as board director and subsequently elected as president of the American Society for Pharmacy Law. Dr. Horn received a B.S. in pharmacy from the Massachusetts College of Pharmacy and Health Sciences University and is currently a master's degree candidate at the University of Florida College of Pharmacy's Pharmaceutical Outcomes and Policy Program, focusing on patient safety and medication risk management.

Ed Israelski, Ph.D., CHFP, is a consultant and the recently retired director of Human Factors at AbbVie Inc., a biopharmaceutical company. After he joined the company in 2001, he led a cross-company team to imbed best practice human factors engineering (HFE) design methods into all of AbbVie's products, to ensure safety and usability. He did this through hands-on design and evaluation of key new products, managing a group of human factors (HF) professionals; training and mentoring internal resources; writing corporate policy and guidelines; and facilitating the use of outside professional HFE resources. He is the co-convener for International Electrotechnical Commission and International Organization for Standardization Ergonomic and Usability Engineering groups in developing international HF/Usability medical devices standards. Dr. Israelski is also past co-chair of the Association for the Advancement of Medical Instrumentation's Human Factors Engineering Committee, which develops HF standards for medical devices. He is a certified human factors professional (CHFP). He has authored 14 book chapters and numerous articles in the area of HF. He holds 30 patents. He is a Fellow of the Human Factors and Ergonomics Society and a member of the National Academies of Sciences, Engineering, and Medicine's Board on Human-System Integration. He is on the editorial board for the journal *Human Factors* and serves as a regular reviewer for several other scientific journals.

Dr. Israelski has worked as a systems engineer, product manager, market researcher, industrial/organizational psychologist as well as a human factors engineer at various companies, including Lucent Technologies-Bell Labs, formerly AT&T, Ameritech/SBC, and Human Factors International. He is an adjunct instructor at Northwestern University. He received a B.S. in electrical engineering from the New Jersey Institute of Technology, an M.S. in operations research from Columbia University, and a Ph.D. in industrial and engineering psychology from the Stevens Institute of Technology.

Brian Jack, M.D., is professor and chair of the Department of Family Medicine at the Boston University (BU) School of Medicine and Boston Medical Center. Dr. Jack graduated from the University of Massachusetts Medical School and completed his residency training at Brown University. He completed a fellowship at the University of Washington. Dr. Jack came to BU in 1997 as the founding vice chair of the Department of Family Medicine. He has authored more than 130 peer-reviewed articles or book chapters, reviewed papers for major medical journals, and served on health-related grant review panels. He is currently principal investigator on a number of other grants.

His research team has developed the Reengineered Discharge Program (Project RED), adapted by the National Quality Forum as a national safe practice. RED is being used in all states and in more than 10 countries. He has completed projects with funding from the Agency for Healthcare Research and Quality (AHRQ), including Reengineering the Hospital Discharge for Patient Safety, which provided an in-depth analysis of the hospital discharge process. RED was then tested in Testing the Re-Engineered Hospital Discharge, a randomized controlled trial funded by AHRQ in the Partners in Patient Safety grants.

He received the 2013 Peter F. Drucker Award for Non-Profit Innovation, the Patient Care Award for Excellence in Patent Education Innovation award, the AHRQ Patient Safety Investigator award, and the Best Research Paper of the Year award of the Society of Teachers of Family Medicine. He was selected to *HealthLeaders* magazine's annual "People Who Make Healthcare Better" list and one of Boston's "Best Doctors" each year from 2010 2015. His *Annals of Internal Medicine* article describing RED is listed in the book *50 Studies Every Physician Should Know*. In 2013 he was elected to the National Academy of Medicine. Dr. Jack has also been active in the worldwide development of family medicine. He is director of the Lesotho Boston Health Alliance, a Kellogg Foundation–funded program that aims to improve the quality of district health services in Lesotho. He is a founding member of the American Academy of Family Physicians Center for International Initiatives. He spent a sabbatical year in Budapest, Hungary, in 1995 where he received a special citation from the mayor of Budapest. He taught in Jordan and Pakistan and has worked on the development of family medicine in Albania, Jordan, Lesotho, Romania, and Vietnam.

Charles Lee, M.D., has been a leading national advocate for simplifying and making medical information more understandable for patients. Dr. Lee is founder and president of Polyglot Systems (Morrisville, North Carolina), built with a mission to develop practical, affordable multilanguage technology solutions to improve health care access and reduce disparities for underserved and limited English-proficient patient populations. He is an internal medicine physician and past National Library of Medicine fellow in medical informatics at the University of North Carolina (UNC) at Chapel Hill/Duke University. He has extensive experience in patient-centered health care communication, language barriers, health literacy, health care software user experience, and instructional design. He is also an adjunct assistant professor at the UNC Eshelman School of Pharmacy, where he is working on several projects to improve medication adherence. Dr. Lee is also a member of the U.S. Food and Drug Administration's Risk Communication Advisory Committee and the Duke Clinical Research Institute's Medication Adherence Alliance, and co-chair of Workgroup for Electronic Date Interchange's Care Coordination Workgroup.

Joan Guthrie Medlen, M.Ed., RDN, LN, is a registered dietitian with an advanced certificate in Adult Weight Management from the American Dietetic Association. She has a master's in education with a focus on instruction design and an interest in universal design for learning, especially for people with intellectual disabilities who are nonverbal and who have trouble writing. Ms. Medlen is the author of *The Down Syndrome Nutrition Handbook: A Guide to Promoting Healthy Lifestyles* (2002, 2006), the first, and only, text dedicated to promoting healthy living for people with Down syndrome of any age. Ms. Medlen focuses her wide array of activities on nutrition and wellness coaching for people of all ages and stages.

Darvece A. Monson is the CEO and founder of More Than Your Kidneys. In 2015, at 34 years old, Ms. Monson founded More Than Your Kidneys at her hospital bedside table with $50 and a refurbished computer. A lifelong "health nut," the nurse of 18 years had been diagnosed with chronic kidney disease, followed by heart failure, severe anemia, end-stage renal disease, and hemodialysis over the years. Ms. Monson is now a kidney transplant candidate. She is well known for her tireless dedication to the aforementioned causes via her personal testimonies and vigor for life. Her innovative work in transforming the world's understanding of kidney survivorship continues to pave the way for survivors across the country. Her education, professional development, and life experience spans a variety of interests. It includes various acclaimed credentials from Lewis University, Moraine Valley Community College, University of Illinois, and BLUE1647.

Ms. Monson has solidified partnerships with the National Kidney Foundation, and participated in clinician forums as well as patient advocacy panels and informational sessions. She has also solidified partnerships with American Funds, and participated in community health promotion, screening, and education efforts as a Certified Kidney Educator through the American Kidney Fund. Her most recent endeavors include being appointed as a member and patient liaison of the National Kidney Foundation Kidney Advocacy Committee, as well as the National Kidney Foundation Associate Board. Her organization has received several awards for helping others obtain funding, grants, and training; eradicate student loans; and advocate for tenant and employer disability rights. Ms. Monson was the September 2016 "Elevate" Feature in *Ebony Magazine*, in which she discussed dialysis, kidney survivorship, three-dimensional kidney transplantation, and making an impact by encouraging awareness, education, and participation.

Dan Morrow, Ph.D., is a professor and chair of the Department of Educational Psychology at the University of Illinois at Urbana-Champaign, with appointments in the Beckman Institute of Advanced Science and Technology and the Departments of Psychology and Industrial and Enterprise Engineering. His research on the impact of aging on cognition, communication, and decision making in the health care domain (health literacy and comprehension of self-care information) and in the aviation domain (air–ground communication; pilot decision making) has been funded by the National Institutes of Health, Agency for Healthcare Research and Quality, Federal Aviation Administration, and National Aeronautics and Space Administration. He is past president of Division 21 of the American Psychological Association (Applied Experimental and Engineering Psychology) and is a fellow of the American Psychological Association and the Human Factors and Ergonomics Society. He has served on advisory committees for the U.S. Food and Drug Administration and the U.S. Pharmacopeial Convention. He is also an incoming editor of the *Journal of Experimental Psychology: Applied*. He received a Ph.D. in cognitive psychology from the University of California, Berkeley, and was a postdoctoral fellow at Stanford University.

Laurie Myers, M.B.A., has led health literacy strategy for Merck Sharp & Dohme Corp. (Merck) since 2011, recently expanding her role to have both U.S. and global responsibility. She focuses on the integration of health literacy externally and across divisions at Merck. Key projects include patient labeling, packaging, clinical trials, and patient education. She has regularly engaged with payers, integrated health systems, and large medical groups to discuss health literacy. Besides serving on the Health Literacy Roundtable, Ms. Myers actively participates on several external projects, including as co-chair of the Harvard Multi-Regional Clinical Trials Center

Return of Results Group; European Medicines Agency lay summaries working group; and as part of the Walgreens/Northwestern/Alliance of Chicago partnership, measuring the impact of the Universal Medication Schedule on patient adherence and health. She is passionate about creating health literacy champions outside of the field and hence speaks at conferences focused in other areas, including adherence, patient engagement and advocacy, market research, Drug Information Association, and lay summaries, in both the United States and Europe. Ms. Myers joined Merck in 1999 and has worked in several therapeutic areas in market research, marketing communications, and pharmacy and distribution. She received her M.B.A. in health care management from the Wharton School at the University of Pennsylvania and graduated magna cum laude with her B.A. in psychology from Yale University.

Terri Ann Parnell, D.N.P., M.A., RN, FAAN, is a nurse, a nationally recognized health literacy expert, and an award-winning author. She is principal and founder of Health Literacy Partners, a corporation that specializes in providing a tapestry of solutions to promote health equity by enhancing person-centered care, effective communication, and the patient experience. Her recent experience includes providing health literacy education and consultation to several New York State Delivery System Reform Incentive Payment Program Performing Provider Systems. Previously, Dr. Parnell was vice president for Health Literacy and Patient Education for the Northwell Health System, where she was responsible for the health literacy strategic plan and integrating concepts of health literacy, language access services, and cultural awareness into core activities across the system.

Dr. Parnell is a member of the National Academies of Sciences, Engineering, and Medicine's Roundtable on Health Literacy and has served as a committee member on the American Nurses Association Care Coordination Quality Measures Panel. She is a fellow in the American Academy of Nursing and The New York Academy of Medicine and has been selected for the 2016/17 The New York Academy of Medicine Fellow Ambassadors Program. In 2016, Dr. Parnell joined TVR Communications Advisory Board as its chief nursing officer. Her second book, *Health Literacy in Nursing: Providing Person-Centered Care*, received an *American Journal of Nursing* 2015 Book of the Year Award in the category of Nursing Management and Leadership. Dr. Parnell is a graduate of St. Vincent's Hospital School of Nursing in New York City. She earned a B.S. in nursing from Adelphi University, a master's degree in health care administration from Hofstra University, and a doctor of nursing practice degree from Case Western Reserve University.

Bobbie Reed is the concerned mother of an adult child who has experienced end-stage renal disease (ESRD) and, in November 2015, a kidney transplant. She has worked as a customer service representative in commercial accounts for Bell of Pennsylvania. Later she worked at AT&T, where she remained for more than 20 years. Her life changed radically when, in May 2013, her son Alex became extremely ill. He was diagnosed with ESRD that October; by December, he began dialysis as a home hemodialysis patient. In November 2015, Alex received a kidney transplant from a non-relative living donor. Along with reaching out to multiple business and professional affiliates, Ms. Reed has become active with the Kidney Health Initiative (KHI). While attending a KHI meeting, she told her family's story of kidney disease in a taped interview for the American Society of Nephrology, which presented the tape at its national meeting. She is also a member of the American Association of Kidney Patients and has attended its national meeting in Nashville, Tennessee, for the past 2 years. Ms. Reed has successfully reached out to Pennsylvania state legislators to request their support in raising awareness about the importance of organ donation, specifically drawing attention to her son's need for a transplant. She has also traveled with the National Kidney Foundation as its Pennsylvania Kidney Advocacy Committee Liaison and called on her legislators to lobby for better laws for the protection and improvement of care of transplant patients and donors. She attended Indiana University of Pennsylvania and obtained a B.S. from the School of Home Economics, studying consumer services with a concentration in business and economics.

Heather Rennie, J.D., is a managing counsel in the regulatory legal group of Merck Sharp & Dohme Corp., a subsidiary of Merck & Co., Inc. Ms. Rennie joined Merck in 2005. During her tenure at Merck, she has provided regulatory legal support for a variety of prescription products and vaccines. She currently supports Merck's diabetes franchise, and serves as the regulatory legal point for product labeling. Prior to joining Merck, Ms. Rennie was a litigation partner with Eckert Seamans Cherin & Mellott, LLC, where she handled a broad range of litigation matters. She earned a B.A. from the College of William and Mary, and graduated cum laude from the Dickinson School of Law at Pennsylvania State University, where she was a member of the *Dickinson Law Review*.

Caleb Sexton has 9 years of experience as a designer, researcher, and strategist. He has worked with large and small teams on strategic innovation for technology start-ups, communities, universities, large government agencies, and Fortune 500 corporations. Throughout this time, his work has included product and service design, management, market and organizational strategy, new market development, and deep-dive contextual research. He has an extensive background in project management, design research, and ethnographic practices that have investigated consumer behavior and habits and translated them into the design of new product and service offerings for organizations and institutions. As a project manager, Mr. Sexton has led design, strategy, and research teams from discovery to development to implementation of new offerings, findings, or strategies that leverage the human-centered design (HCD) process. Over the past 2 years, his efforts have focused on health care technology research and how HCD can bring innovative opportunities to early-stage discovery and development. As a psoriatic patient himself, he has a deeply vested interest in empowering and enabling better care management for others with psoriatic disease. This has led to his interest into exploring ways that design, technology, and strategy can be aligned to help facilitate better care and communication between patients and their care providers while supporting the psoriatic disease research community.

William Shrank, M.D., M.S., joined the University of Pittsburgh Medical Center's (UPMC's) Health Plan Division in June 2016 as the company's new chief medical officer. In this role, Dr. Shrank will focus on the design and implementation of new payment and delivery models to promote improved population health and further advance UPMC's integrated clinical business strategies.

Prior to joining UPMC, Dr. Shrank served as senior vice president, chief scientific officer, and chief medical officer of provider innovation for CVS Health, where he led the development of solutions to support providers to manage risk and deliver better care for the populations they serve. Prior to joining CVS, Dr. Shrank served as the inaugural director, Research and Rapid-Cycle Evaluation for the Center for Medicare & Medicaid Innovation at the Centers for Medicare & Medicaid Services (CMS), where he helped design and led the evaluation of new payment reform models tested by the center such as pioneer accountable care organizations, bundled payments, and progressive primary care models. Dr. Shrank began his career as a practicing physician with Brigham Internal Medicine Associates at Brigham and Women's Hospital in Boston, as well as an assistant professor at Harvard Medical School. His research at Harvard focused on improving the quality of prescribing and the use of chronic medications, and he published nearly 200 papers on these topics.

Dr. Shrank has served on various national committees and advisory boards related to health. Among the many achievement awards Dr. Shrank received is the 2015 Healthcare Executive Transformation Award from the Los Angeles County Medical Association. He also was the recipient of the Robert Wood Johnson Foundation Pioneer Award to evaluate the effect of innovative prescription label design on adherence to chronic medication and health outcomes. Dr. Shrank received his M.D. from Cornell University Medical College, served his residency in internal medicine at Georgetown

University, and was a Fellow in Health Policy Research at the University of California, Los Angeles (UCLA), RAND. He earned his M.S. in health services from UCLA and his bachelor's degree from Brown University.

Steve Sparks, M.A., provides leadership for Wisconsin Health Literacy, a division of Wisconsin Literacy, Inc., a statewide nonprofit organization. He provides consultation and coordination for statewide health literacy strategies and programs for health and social service organizations and for the public. Mr. Sparks has spent his career in health and health care communication. Before joining Wisconsin Health Literacy, he held marketing, communications, and fundraising positions in four hospitals and health systems in Iowa, Nebraska, and Wisconsin. Most recently he was regional director of marketing and public relations for SSM Health Care of Wisconsin. He has taught communications courses at the University of Wisconsin–Madison, Madison College, and the University of Nebraska. He is a certified Toastmaster and the first recipient of the local Public Relations Society of America Communicator of the Year award. Mr. Sparks has conducted numerous health literacy training sessions with health care and health insurance professionals and led several health literacy interventions on public health issues. He currently leads a project funded through the Advancing a Healthier Wisconsin Endowment of the Medical College of Wisconsin. The goal of the project is to implement easier-to-understand prescription medication labels in Wisconsin. He has been a presenter at several national health literacy conferences, including the Wisconsin Health Literacy Summit, which he coordinates. He holds a bachelor's degree in English education and a master's degree in journalism and mass communication.

Elisabeth Walther, Pharm.D., J.D., is a health scientist policy analyst at the U.S. Food and Drug Administration, where she currently leads regulatory policy development related to patient prescription drug product information. She also continues to practice as a community pharmacist. She holds a Pharm.D. and a J.D. from Drake University.

Michael Wolf, Ph.D., M.A., M.P.H., is a professor of medicine, associate division chief (Internal Medicine and Geriatrics), and director of the Health Literacy & Learning Program (HeLP) within the Feinberg School of Medicine, Northwestern University. He also holds appointments in the Departments of Cognitive Sciences, Communication Studies, Medical Social Sciences, Psychiatry and Behavioral Sciences, and Surgery. As a health services researcher and cognitive-behavioral scientist, Dr. Wolf has extensively studied cognitive, psychosocial, and health system determinants of health, specifically in the areas of health literacy and health communications research. His work has focused primarily on understanding health care complexity. Dr. Wolf has led several large-scale, pragmatic trials to evaluate multifaceted interventions to promote patient engagement in health, targeting chronic disease self-management, medication safety, and adherence.

H. Shonna Yin, M.D., M.Sc., is a general pediatrician and an assistant professor of pediatrics and population health at the New York University School of Medicine/Bellevue Hospital Center. She is a National Institutes of Health (NIH)-funded researcher whose work centers on the issue of health literacy and its implications for child health. A large focus of her work involves examining the intersection between health literacy and medication safety, including the development and evaluation of low-literacy strategies to improve parent understanding of medication instructions. Dr. Yin is principal investigator of a multisite R01 funded by Eunice Kennedy Shriver National Institute of Child Health and Human Development (NICHD) to develop and evaluate a low-literacy medication labeling and dosing strategy for pediatric prescription liquid medications. Some of her work in medication safety is featured in the Joint Commission book *Addressing Patients' Health Literacy Needs*. Dr. Yin is a key member of the Centers for Disease Control and Prevention's (CDC's) PROTECT (Prevention of Overdoses and Treatment Errors in Children Taskforce) initiative, and served as co-chair of the subcommittee focused on the standardization of pediatric medication dosing instructions. She also serves as a member of the U.S. Food and Drug Administration's (FDA's) Risk Communication Advisory Committee. Other areas of research focus include examining low-literacy strategies to address obesity prevention as well as chronic disease management (e.g., asthma). Dr. Yin serves as co-principal investigator of a multisite NIH/NICHD-funded R01 to develop and test a low-literacy and numeracy-focused intervention for early childhood obesity prevention (Greenlight). She is also working on a Clinical Translational Science Institute–funded project to improve health provider and parent management of child asthma through a health literacy, information technology–based approach. Dr. Yin has provided health literacy expertise to many groups, including CDC; FDA; the National Academies of Sciences, Engineering, and Medicine; and the American Academy of Pediatrics. She was a Robert Wood Johnson Foundation Physician Faculty Scholar (2009-2012), and recipient of the Pfizer Fellowship in Health Literacy/Clear Health Communication (2007-2009).